DVD Contents

OPERATIVETECHNIQUES

hip arthritis
surgery

OPERATIVE TECHNIQUES

hip arthritis
surgery

James P. Waddell, MD, FRCSC
Professor, Division of Orthopaedic Surgery
University of Toronto
Staff Surgeon, St. Michael's Hospital
Head, Holland Orthopaedic & Arthritic Centre
Toronto, Ontario, Canada

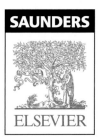

SAUNDERS

ELSEVIER

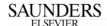

1600 John F. Kennedy Blvd.
Ste 1800
Philadelphia, PA 19103-2899

OPERATIVE TECHNIQUES: HIP ARTHRITIS SURGERY　　　　　ISBN: 978-1-4160-3850-4

Notice

Knowledge and best practice in this field are constantly changing. As new research and experience broaden our knowledge, changes in practice, treatment and drug therapy may become necessary or appropriate. Readers are advised to check the most current information provided (i) on procedures featured or (ii) by the manufacturer of each product to be administered, to verify the recommended dose or formula, the method and duration of administration, and contraindications. It is the responsibility of the practitioner, relying on their own experience and knowledge of the patient, to make diagnoses, to determine dosages and the best treatment for each individual patient, and to take all appropriate safety precautions. To the fullest extent of the law, neither the Publisher nor the Editor assumes any liability for any injury and/or damage to persons or property arising out or related to any use of the material contained in this book.

The Publisher

Library of Congress Cataloging-in-Publication Data
Waddell, J. P. (James P.)
　　Operative techniques : hip arthritis surgery / James P. Waddell.—1st ed.
　　　　p. ; cm.
　　Includes index.
　　ISBN 978-1-4160-3850-4
1. Hip–Surgery–Handbooks, manuals, etc.　2. Arthritis–Surgery–Handbooks, manuals, etc.
3. Total hip replacement–Handbooks, manuals, etc.　I. Title.
　　[DNLM: 1. Arthroplasty, Replacement, Hip–methods–Handbooks.　2. Arthritis–surgery–
Handbooks.　3. Osteotomy–methods–Handbooks.　4. Reoperation–methods–Handbooks.
WE 39 W116o 2008]
　　RD549.W27 2008
　　617.5'81059—dc22　　　　　　　　　　　　　　　　　　2008004401

Publishing Director: Kimberly Murphy
Design Direction: Steven Stave

Printed in China

Last digit is the print number:　9　8　7　6　5　4　3　2　1

CONTRIBUTORS

Paul E. Beaulé, MD, FRCSC
Associate Professor, University of Ottawa; Head,
    Adult Reconstruction, The Ottawa Hospital,
    Ottawa, Ontario, Canada
    Hip Resurfacing Arthroplasty

Petros J. Boscainos, MD
Orthopaedic Clinical Fellow, University of Toronto,
    and Toronto East General Hospital; Research
    Fellow, Mount Sinai Hospital, Toronto, Ontario,
    Canada
    Rings and Cages

Robert B. Bourne, MD, FRCSC
Professor, Orthopaedic Surgery, University of
    Western Ontario, and London Health Sciences
    Centre, London, Ontario, Canada
    Direct Lateral Exposure

John A. F. Charity, MD
Robin Ling Hip Fellow, Princess Elizabeth
    Orthopaedic Centre, Royal Devon and
    Exeter NHS Foundation Trust, Exeter, Devon,
    United Kingdom
    Femoral Revision: Impaction Grafting

J. Roderick Davey, MD, FRCS(C)
Associate Professor, Department of Surgery,
    University of Toronto; Associate Director, Surgical
    Services, Head, Division of Orthopaedic Surgery,
    and Medical Director, Toronto Western Operating
    Rooms, University Health Network, Toronto,
    Ontario, Canada
    Direct Lateral Approach to the Hip

John H. Franklin, MD
Assistant Professor, Medical College of Georgia;
    Augusta Orthopaedics, Augusta, Georgia
    The Cemented Femoral Stem

**Graham A. Gie, MB, ChB, FRCS,
FRCSEd(Orth)**
Consultant Orthopaedic Surgeon, Princess Elizabeth
    Orthopaedic Centre, Royal Devon and
    Exeter NHS Foundation Trust, Exeter, Devon,
    United Kingdom
    Femoral Revision: Impaction Grafting

Allan E. Gross, MD, FRCSC
Professor of Surgery, Faculty of Medicine, University
    of Toronto; Orthopaedic Surgeon, Division of
    Orthopaedic Surgery, Mount Sinai Hospital,
    Toronto, Ontario, Canada
    Rings and Cages

**Mahmoud A. Hafez, MSc Orth, Dip SICOT,
FRCS Ed, MD**
Head of the Orthopaedic Department, Division of
    Surgery, Medical School, October 6 University,
    Cairo, Egypt; Formerly Arthroplasty Fellow, St.
    Michael's Hospital, University of Toronto, Toronto,
    Ontario, Canada
    **Templating for Primary Total Hip Arthroplasty;
        Digital Templating for Revision Total Hip
        Arthroplasty**

William J. Hart, MBBS, FRCS(Trauma & Orth)
Consultant Orthopaedic Surgeon, New Cross
    Hospital, Wolverhampton, United Kingdom
    The Cemented Acetabular Component

John P. Hodgkinson, MB, ChB, FRCS(Eng)
Honorary Lecturer Orthopaedics, University of
    Manchester, Manchester; Consultant Orthopaedic
    Surgeon, Washington Hospital, Wigan, Lancashire,
    United Kingdom
    The Cemented Acetabular Component

James L. Howard, MD
Adult Reconstruction Fellow, Mayo Clinic, Rochester,
    Minnesota
    **Minimally Invasive Total Hip Arthroplasty:
        Techniques and Results**

Oliver Keast-Butler, MBChB, FRCS(Orth)
Consultant Orthopaedic Surgeon, Conquest
    Hospital, Hastings, United Kingdom
    **Posterior Approach to the Hip; Femoral Stem
        Revision: Posterior Approach**

**Catherine F. Kellett, BSc(Hons), BM BCH,
FRCS(Tr & Orth)**
Orthopaedic Clinical Fellow, University of Toronto,
    and Mount Sinai Hospital, Toronto, Ontario,
    Canada
    Rings and Cages

Winston Y. Kim, MB, BCh, FRCS(Orth)
Former Fellow, Department of Orthopaedics,
University of British Columbia, Vancouver, British
Columbia, Canada
Acetabular Cementless Revision

Jeremy S. Kudera, MD
Senior Resident, Mayo Clinic, Rochester, Minnesota
**Minimally Invasive Total Hip Arthroplasty:
Techniques and Results**

Jo-ann Lee, MS
Nurse Practitioner, Massachusetts General Hospital,
Harvard University, Boston, and Newton Wellesley
Hospital, Newton, Massachusetts
Hip Arthroscopy

Steven J. MacDonald, MD, FRCS(C)
Associate Professor, Division of Orthopaedic Surgery,
Department of Surgery, University of Western
Ontario; Chief of Orthopaedics and Chief of
Surgery, University Hospital, London, Ontario,
Canada
Cementless Femoral Stems

Henrik Malchau, MD, PhD
Associate Professor of Orthopedics, Harvard Medical
School; Co-Director, Harris Orthopedic
Biomechanics and Biomaterials Lab, and Attending
Physician, Department of Orthopedics,
Massachusetts General Hospital, Boston,
Massachusetts
The Cemented Femoral Stem

Bassam A. Masri, MD, FRCSC
Professor and Chairman, Department of
Orthopaedics, University of British Columbia;
Head, Department of Orthopaedics, Vancouver
Acute Health Services, Vancouver, British
Columbia, Canada
Acetabular Cementless Revision

Wadih Y. Matar, MSc, MD
PGY-5 Resident Orthopaedic Surgery Division,
Department of Surgery, University of Ottawa, and
The Ottawa Hospital, Ottawa, Ontario, Canada
Hip Resurfacing Arthroplasty

Joseph C. McCarthy, MD
Vice Chairman, Department of Orthopaedic Surgery,
Massachusetts General Hospital, Harvard
University; Director, Center for Joint Reconstructive
Surgery, Newton Wellesley Hospital, Newton,
Massachusetts
Hip Arthroscopy

Michael B. Millis, MD
Associate Professor of Clinical Orthopaedic Surgery,
Harvard Medical School; Director, Adolescent and
Young Adult Hip Unit, Children's Hospital Boston,
Boston, Massachusetts
Bernese Periacetabular Osteotomy

Wayne G. Paprosky, MD
Associate Professor, Orthopaedic Surgery,
Rush University Medical Center, Chicago;
Attending Physician, Central DuPage Hospital,
Winfield, Illinois
**Extended Trochanteric Osteotomy:
Posterior Approach**

Michael D. Ries, MD
Professor of Orthopaedic Surgery, and Chief of
Arthroplasty, University of California, San
Francisco, San Francisco, California
Cementless Acetabular Cup Technique

Emil H. Schemitsch, MD, FRCS(C)
Professor of Orthopaedics, and Head, Division of
Orthopaedic Surgery, Department of Surgery, St.
Michael's Hospital, University of Toronto, Toronto,
Ontario, Canada
**Templating for Primary Total Hip Arthroplasty;
Digital Templating for Revision Total Hip
Arthroplasty**

Scott M. Sporer, MD, MS
Associate Professor, Orthopaedic Surgery,
Rush University Medical Center, Chicago;
Attending Physician, Central DuPage Hospital,
Winfield, Illinois
**Extended Trochanteric Osteotomy: Posterior
Approach**

A. John Timperley, MB, ChB, FRCSEd, DPhil
Consultant Orthopaedic Surgeon,
Princess Elizabeth Orthopaedic Centre, Royal
Devon and Exeter NHS Foundation Trust, Exeter,
Devon, United Kingdom
Femoral Revision: Impaction Grafting

Robert T. Trousdale, MD
Professor of Orthopedics, Mayo Clinic, Rochester,
Minnesota
**Minimally Invasive Total Hip Arthroplasty:
Techniques and Results**

Nezar S. Tumia, MBBCh, FRCS(Tr&Orth), MD
Fellow in Orthopaedic Surgery, St. Michael's
Hospital, Toronto, Ontario, Canada
Intertrochanteric Femoral Osteotomy

James P. Waddell, MD, FRCSC
Professor, Division of Orthopaedic Surgery,
    University of Toronto; Staff Surgeon, St. Michael's
    Hospital; Head, Holland Orthopaedic & Arthritic
    Centre, Toronto, Ontario, Canada
    **Intertrochanteric Femoral Osteotomy; Posterior
    Approach to the Hip; Femoral Stem Revision:
    Posterior Approach**

**Claire F. Young, MB, ChB,
FRCS(Tr & Orth)**
Consultant Orthopaedic Surgeon, Cumberland
    Infirmary, Carlisle, United Kingdom
    Cementless Femoral Stems

PREFACE

Adult hip surgery occupies a special role in orthopedic surgery. Early orthopedic practitioners recognized the disabling effects of hip arthritis, and many of the earliest orthopedic efforts were designed to address this crippling problem. Osteotomy, partial joint replacement, interposition arthroplasty, and finally total joint replacement were all pioneered in the treatment of adult hip disease.

With increasing knowledge of the relationship between structural abnormality of the hip based on congenital deformity or childhood illness and adult hip arthritis, surgical procedures designed to correct these underlying malformations were promoted in the expectation that treatment of these problems could prevent later onset of significant adult hip arthritis.

As adult hip surgery became more common and more sophisticated, it became evident that the technical component of these surgical procedures was of paramount importance in their success or failure. Therefore, there continues to be increased interest in the technical aspects of hip surgery, recognizing that there is a direct correlation between technical excellence and longevity of the procedure.

For that reason I was delighted when Elsevier asked me to edit a volume on the surgical techniques in adult hip surgery. I felt it was imperative that the chapters in this volume be written by individuals with excellent academic credentials, publications that demonstrated the quality of their clinical outcomes, and a strong desire to teach others the technical aspects of these often challenging surgical procedures.

I have not been disappointed. I believe the production qualities of this volume are of the highest possible standard and that the combination of illustration and text nicely highlights the issues around the surgical procedures described.

I would like to thank all the contributors to this volume for their tremendous effort in making it a success. I would especially like to thank Kimberly Murphy of Elsevier for the concept and direction and Berta Steiner for her firm editorial hand.

It has been a pleasure for me to be associated with this project, and I hope you enjoy the end product.

James P. Waddell, MD, FRCSC

FOREWORD

The advances in treatment for the diseased hip over the last 40 years have been incredibly significant. Not only has hip arthroplasty become one of the most successful procedures ever and continues to get better thanks to the contributions of many, but also over the last decade there has been particularly rapid employment of new bearing materials, designs and a resurgence of hip resurfacing. In addition, non-arthroplasty approaches for the hip with arthropathy have evolved with a definite role in postponing the need for prosthetic intervention.

Professor James Waddell has herewith added his contribution to the education of the many who are interested in these disciplines by assembling an excellent volume which includes the most important, established techniques used today presented by very knowledgeable and experienced hip reconstructive surgeons. Doctor Waddell was well-suited to the task of assembling the fine points of these techniques because of his long experience with reconstructive surgery of the lower extremity and his long devotion to education that has culminated in his position as Chairman, Division of Orthopaedic Surgery, Department of Surgery at the University of Toronto. The chapter's strong points are the very clear and concise stepwise instructions and the beautifully illustrated techniques with key references which will be of great value to students, PA's, residents, fellows and even patients, who in this modern day of the internet often desire to know "everything" about treatment options for their maladies and particularly arthritis of their hips.

Harlan C. Amstutz, MD
Emeritus Professor
Orthopaedic Surgery
UCLA School of Medicine
Medical Director
Joint Replacement Institute
St. Vincent Medical Center
Los Angeles, California

CONTENTS

Non–Joint Replacement Surgery

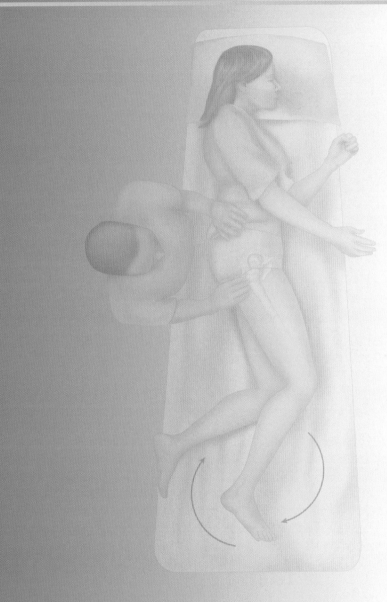

Hip Arthroscopy

Joseph C. McCarthy and Jo-ann Lee

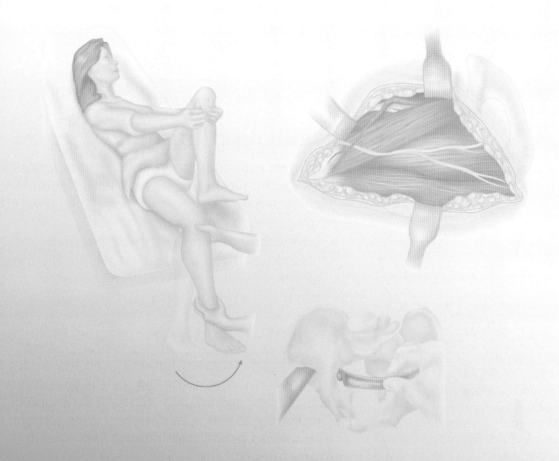

Controversies

- Morbid obesity is a relative contraindication for arthroscopy, not only because of distraction limitations but also because of the requisite length of instruments necessary to access and maneuver within the deeply recessed joint.
- Moderate dysplasia needs to be judiciously evaluated prior to arthroscopic intervention.
- Candidates for hip arthroscopy should have reproducible symptoms and physical findings that limit function, along with a history of mechanical symptoms such as clicking, catching, locking, or buckling.

Treatment Options

- Lateral approach
- Supine approach

Indications

- Labral tears
- Chondral lesions
- Loose bodies
- Synovial diseases: synovial chondromatosis, pigmented villonodular synovitis
- Trauma
- Crystalline diseases (gout, pseudogout)
- Previous total hip arthroplasty
- Early-stage osteonecrosis
- Symptomatic impingement

Examination/Imaging

- Positive examination findings include a positive McCarthy sign; inguinal pain with flexion, adduction, and internal rotation; and inguinal pain with resisted straight leg-raising test.
- Gadolinium-enhanced arthrogram magnetic resonance imaging may increase the diagnostic yield of intra-articular hip pathology, as shown by the labral tear evident in Figure 1 *(arrow)*.

Surgical Anatomy

- The deeply recessed femoral head lies within the bony acetabulum. The hip joint is enclosed within a thick fibrocapsular and muscular envelope in close proximity to the sciatic nerve, lateral femoral cutaneous nerve, and femoral neurovascular structures.
- Fluoroscopic images determine the relative distraction of the femoral head from the acetabulum (see accompanying video).
  - The negative intra-articular pressure that results from the distraction force is released using a 6-inch, 18-gauge spinal needle with a Nytinol wire and an image intensifier if necessary. The needle is placed superior to the greater trochanter and tangential to the acetabulum, and a "give" sensation is felt upon capsule entry.
  - A second 6-inch, 18-gauge spinal needle is then advanced into the hip capsule, and then the joint is injected with approximately 30 to 40 ml of normal saline. Flow from the second spinal needle confirms intra-articular placement of both needles.

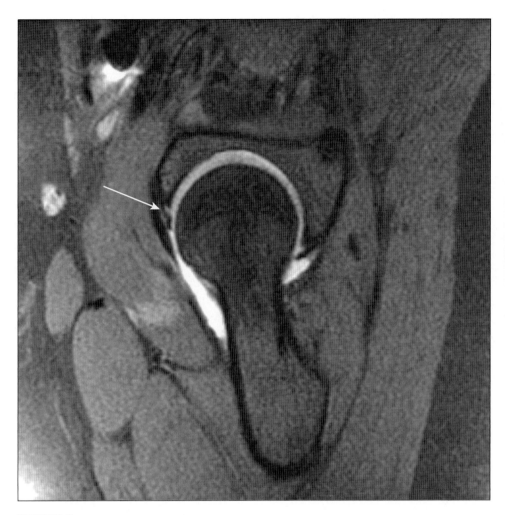

FIGURE 1

Equipment

- Dedicated hip distractor is available through Innomed Corp (Savannah, GA).

Controversies

- Surgeon preference for lateral vs. supine position.

Positioning

- The lateral approach requires that the patient be positioned in the lateral decubitus position with the affected hip up. Most intra-articular lesions occur in the anterior quadrant of the hip and can be treated easily via the two primary portals of the lateral approach. Surgeons may use a modified fracture table, or a dedicated hip distractor can be positioned on a regular operating room table and adjusted in multiple planes (Fig. 2).
- Adequate distraction is required to separate the femoral head away from the acetabulum to allow passage of instruments into the recesses of the joint.
- A well-padded perineal post is positioned and adjusted prior to applying traction.
- Axial traction is applied via a carefully padded foot boot with the heel firmly seated and secured. The traction device is adjusted such that the foot can be maintained in neutral position with respect to eversion and/or inversion of the hindfoot, thereby avoiding undue stress to the ligamentous structures on one side or the other of the ankle.
- Distraction is applied with the leg abducted between 0° and 20°, depending on the patient's neck shaft angle and the depth of the acetabulum. The hip then is placed in slight forward flexion of approximately 10–20°.

Portals/Exposures

- Lateral approach (Fig. 3)
  - The skin incisions are superficial, not penetrating deeper than the subcutaneous adipose tissue. Then, tapered blunt trocars are used to pass through the adipose, fascia, and muscle tissue. This technique protects all interceding neurovascular structures and muscle from sharp equipment and repetitive trauma during the exchange of instruments.
  - The pressure required varies by patient and by capsular location. A lens may be needed.
- Anterior superior paratrochanteric portal
  - The anterior superior paratrochanteric portal provides excellent visualization of the femoral head, anterior neck, anterior labrum, and synovial tissues beneath the zona orbicularis.

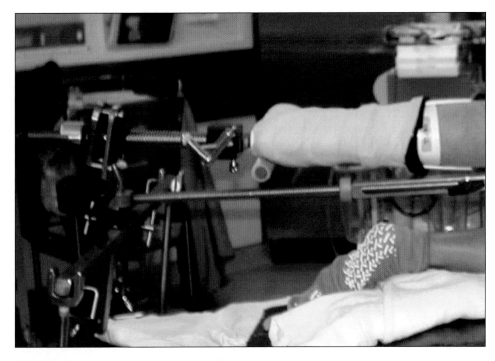

FIGURE 2

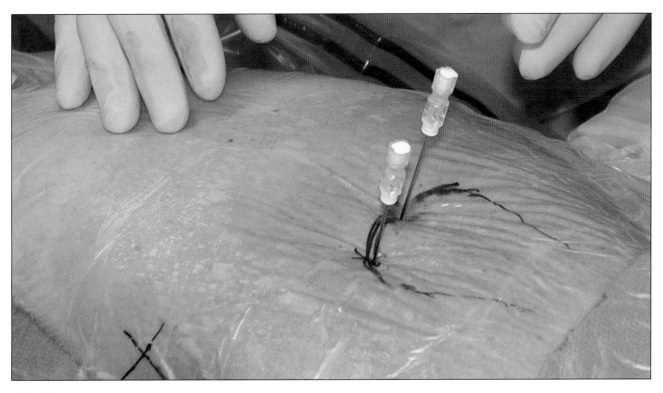

FIGURE 3

PEARLS

- *The paratrochanteric portals pass through fewer muscle planes, avoid potential injury to the lateral femoral cutaneous nerve, and puncture the superior hip capsule, which is slightly thinner.*

- *Image intensification is helpful to alter the position of the portal pathway. The posterolateral portal is considered a very safe portal. Placing this portal under direct visualization facilitates its intra-articular position. This is commonly done by placing the camera in the anterolateral portal first.*

PITFALLS

- *The neurovascular structure that is at potential risk with the anterior superior paratrochanteric portal is the superior gluteal nerve. It is located 4–6 centimeters above the tip of the greater trochanter.*

- *The initial trocar placement for the posterior superior paratrochanteric portal is slightly superior and slightly anterior to avoid deflection posteriorly and potential injury to the sciatic nerve. Positioning of the hip in flexion greater than 20° can translate the sciatic nerve anteriorly, bringing this structure into jeopardy. Likewise, external rotation of the femur posteriorly translates the greater trochanter and increases the likelihood of posterior deflection of the trocar, which may potentiate injury to the sciatic nerve. It is for this reason that the leg must be placed in neutral or slight internal rotation when passing the needle or trocar for this portal.*

In combination with the posterior superior trochanteric portal, it is an extremely useful portal for instrumentation and treatment of anterior labral lesions and acetabular chondral lesions.

- The cannula is aimed toward the center of the acetabulum at the fovea while keeping it as close to the femoral head as possible.
- This portal transgresses the anterior musculotendinous junction of the gluteus medius, the tendinous region of the gluteus minimus, and the anterior hip capsule before entering the joint.

■ Posterior superior paratrochanteric portal

- The posterior paratrochanteric portal is used to view the posterior capsule, posterior labrum, and the posterior femoral head.

Instrumentation

- The intra-articular structures in the hip joint can most often be visualized with a standard 30° arthroscope; however, there are times when a 70° arthroscope is benenficial.
- Telescoping cannulas are extremely helpful for removal of large loose bodies or to accommodate angled punches.
- A variety of probes and hooks are first used to evaluate the intra-articular structures.
- A variety of long suction punches have been designed specifically for hip arthroscopy.
- Extra-length mechanical shavers can also be useful for débridement of labral tears.
- Curved shaver blades with either convex or concave surfaces improve navigation of the convex surface of the femoral head.
- An unsheathed bur is helpful should bony resection be necessary.
- Flexible thermal devices with precise control of temperature and coagulation are extremely useful in débriding chondral flaps and the torn labral rim.

Controversies

- An important point with the posterolateral portal is that the "pop" that is encountered when entering the joint must be felt before bone is encountered. If bone is felt without the sensation of traversing the capsule, the trocar is either too high and the outer wall of the acetabulum is encountered, or too low and the head of the femur is encountered.

PEARLS

- *Flexible thermal devices with precise control of temperature and coagulation are extremely useful in débriding chondral flaps and the torn labral rim.*

- *Inflamed, redundant synovial tissue can also be resected and coagulated.*

PITFALLS

- *Over-resection of labral tissue should be avoided.*

- The entry point for this portal is placed at the junction of the posterior and middle thirds of the superior trochanteric ridge, essentially mirroring the anterior paratrochanteric portal.
- Correct positioning of the posterior trochanteric portal passes through the posterior margin of the musculotendinous junction of the gluteus medius muscle.

Procedure

STEP 1

- Have a routine sequence for visualization of the central compartment.
- The labrum is an important anatomic structure in the hip joint with many functions; therefore, the least intrusive means of resecting or stabilizing a labral tear (Fig. 4, *arrow*) should be emphasized.
- Arthroscopic treatment of labral tears involves judicious débridement back to a stable base and to healthy-appearing tissue while preserving the capsular labral tissue.

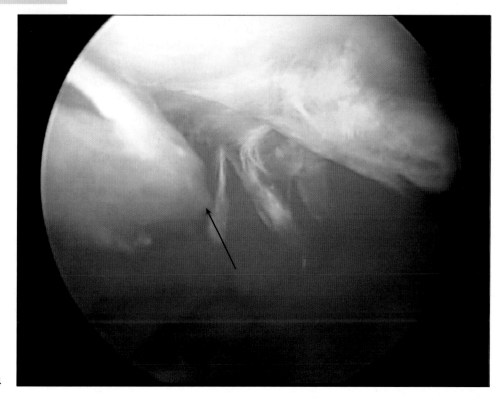

FIGURE 4

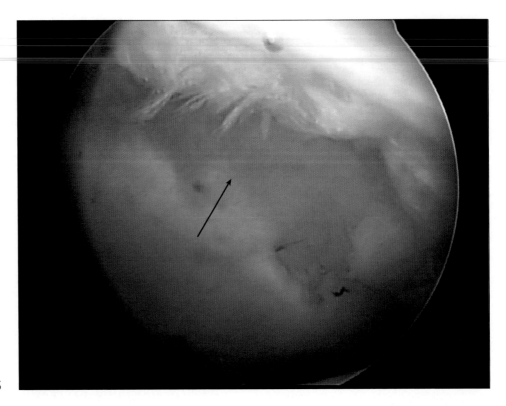

FIGURE 5

Instrumentation/ Implantation

- Labral tears are débrided with straight or curved extra-length shavers.

Instrumentation/ Implantion

- Chondral flaps are addressed using straight and curved shavers, angled basket forceps, and electrothermal tools with straight and flexible tips.
- Microfracture of the chondral lesion may be done with straight or angled picks.

PEARLS

- *The central compartment should be addressed prior to the peripheral compartment.*

STEP 2

- Chondral flaps require chondroplasty. If there is a full-thickness chondral defect (Fig. 5, *arrow*), the subchondral bone is drilled or treated with a microfracture technique to enhance fibrocartilage formation.

STEP 3

- Complete the procedure in the central compartment prior to examining the peripheral compartment.
- If surgery needs to be done in the peripheral compartment, traction is released and the hip is then flexed between 30° and 45°.
- Loose bodies are also sometimes found in the peripheral compartment (Fig. 6, *arrow*), and they can be removed from extra-articular spaces as well using fluoroscopic guidance.

Postoperative Care and Expected Outcomes

- Most patients require crutches from 2 to 7 days. Patients may progress to full weight bearing as soon as comfort allows.
- Most patients are able to drive within 24–48 hours of the surgery.

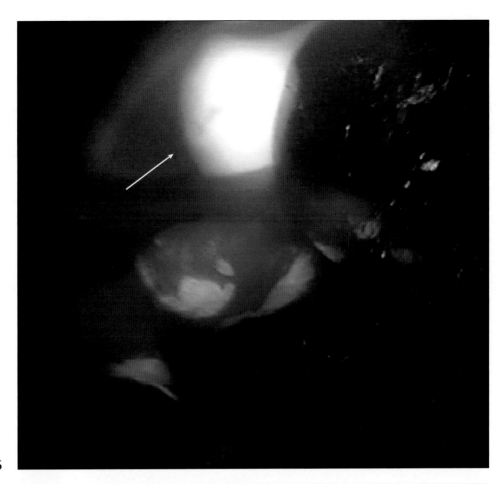

FIGURE 6

Instrumentation/Implantation

- Loose bodies can be resected and simultaneously aspirated with a variety of long suction punches designed specifically for hip arthroscopy.
- Alternatively, a partial synovectomy can be done using straight and curved extra-length shavers.
- Impinging osteophytes can be resected with unhooded burrs under fluoroscopic guidance.

Evidence

Byrd JW. Hip arthroscopy utilizing the supine position. Arthroscopy. 1994;10:275–80.

The supine position in arthroscopic hip surgery is performed on a standard fracture table with fluoroscopy. Traction is used to distract the hip for introduction of the instruments. Three standard arthroscopic portals are routinely used.

Glick JM. Hip arthroscopy using the lateral approach. Instr Course Lect. 1988;37:223–31.

Hip arthroscopy provides complete visualization of the joint space using a direct lateral approach over the greater trochanter, with the patient in the lateral decubitus position. The involved leg is held in an abducted and flexed position with traction by pulleys hung overhead.

McCarthy JC, Lee JA. Acetabular dysplasia: a paradigm of arthroscopic examination of chondral injuries. Clin Orthop. 2002;122–8.

Mild uncovering of the anterior femoral head subjects the labrum to increased load and potential susceptibility to tearing most frequently anteriorly. The findings in the current study support the concept that labral disruption frequently is a predecessor in the continuum of degenerative joint disease.

McCarthy JC, Lee JA. Hip arthroscopy: indications, outcomes, and complications. Instr Course Lect. 2006;55:301–8.

Hip arthroscopy is technically demanding and requires special distraction tools and operating equipment. With proper patient selection hip arthroscopy can successfully manage numerous intra-articular conditions such as labral and chondral injuries, loose bodies, foreign bodies and synovial conditions.

McCarthy JC, Noble PC, Schuck MR, Wright J, Lee J. The Otto E. Aufranc Award: The role of labral lesions to development of early degenerative hip disease. Clin Orthop. 2001;25–37.

Arthroscopic and anatomic observations support the concept that labral disruption and degenerative joint disease are frequently part of a continuum of joint disease.

Intertrochanteric Femoral Osteotomy

Nezar S. Tumia and James P. Waddell

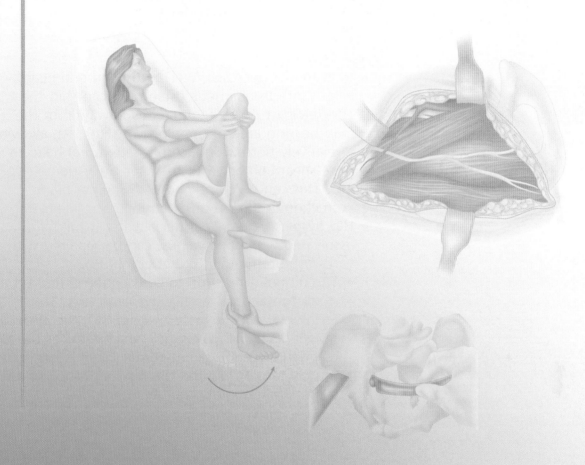

Indications

- Patient selection is crucial for the success of the intertrochanteric osteotomy. Patients should be under the age of 50 years, should be motivated, and should have a clear and realistic understanding of the goal of surgery.
- Various symptomatic hip pathologies can be appropriate indications for intertrochanteric osteotomy.

VARUS OSTEOTOMY

- In avascular necrosis (AVN) of the femoral head, valgus intertrochanteric osteotomy can shift the affected part of the femoral head away from the load-bearing area of the hip joint (Fig. 1A), allowing a relatively normal surface of the femoral head to have shear contact with the acetabular dome (Fig. 1B). This can be combined with sagittal plane correction in flexion or extension.
- Hip dysplasia (Fig. 2), especially if it is mild and associated with coxa valgus, can be repaired with varus osteotomy (Santore et al., 2006).
  - The hip joint reaction force is concentrated on a small contact area in hip dysplasia (Fig. 3A).
  - Following varus osteotomy (Fig. 3B), the abductor muscle lever arm is longer, which reduces the joint reaction force. The joint contact area is larger, and muscle tension around the hip joint is lower due to proximal migration of its insertions.

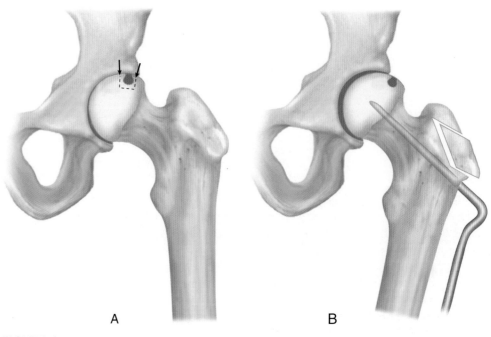

A   B

FIGURE 1

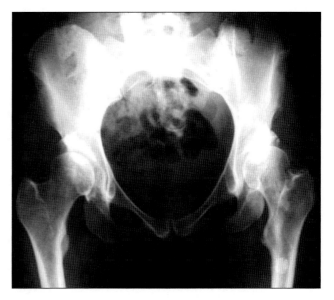

FIGURE 2

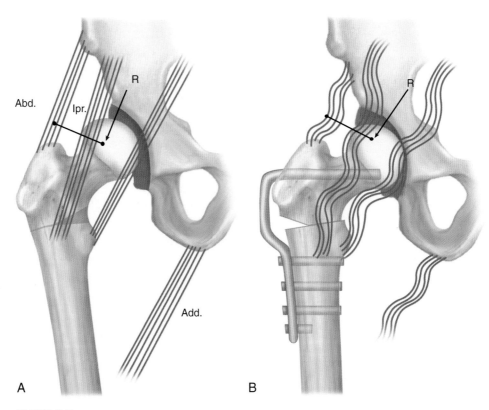

A

B

FIGURE 3

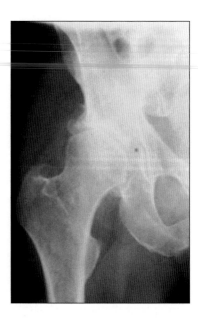

FIGURE 4

■ Pain from focal osteoarthritis can be improved by increasing the abductor lever arm and thereby reducing hip joint reaction force (D'Souza et al., 1998). The degenerative changes should be mild to moderate to achieve better results.
  • The radiograph in Figure 4 shows focal osteoarthritis affecting the hip joint.
  • Careful preoperative planning for a varus intertrochanteric osteotomy (Fig. 5A) resulted in healing of the osteotomy site without distorting the alignment of the intramedullary canal (Fig. 5B).

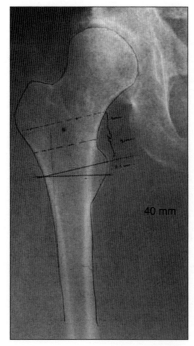
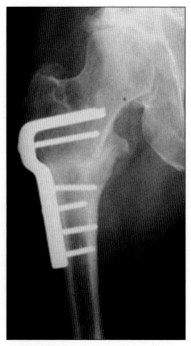

FIGURE 5   A   B

VALGUS OSTEOTOMY

■ Nonunion of a femoral neck fracture can be an indication for valgus intertrochanteric osteotomy, which can change the shear forces across the fractured neck of the femur (Fig. 6A) into compression forces that encourage fracture healing (Fig. 6B).

• The radiograph in Figure 7 shows delayed union of a basal cervical fracture of the proximal femur despite the full reduction and fixation with two screws.

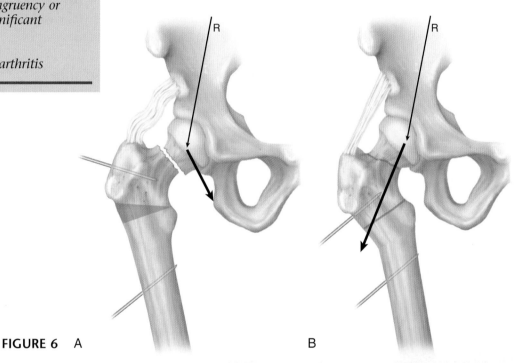

FIGURE 6   A   B

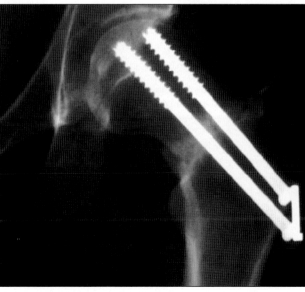

FIGURE 7

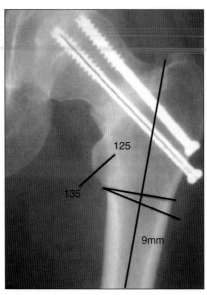 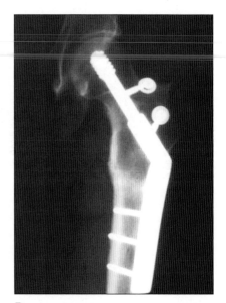

125

135

9mm

FIGURE 8   A   B

- Careful preoperative planning for a valgus intertrochanteric osteotomy (Fig. 8A) resulted in a healed fracture following the osteotomy (Fig. 8B).
■ In Legg-Calvé-Perthes disease, valgus osteotomy can increase leg length and also improve pain when hinge abduction exists.
■ In slipped capital femoral epiphysis, valgus osteotomy, usually combined with flexion correction, can improve pain that results from impingement of the femoral neck against the acetabular rim.

Controversies

- Smoking and obesity might have an adverse effect on the outcome.
- This type of treatment is not ideal for patients engaged in strenuous manual labor or athletes participating in high-impact sports.

Treatment Options

- Femoral osteotomy can be combined with acetabular osteotomy when the main deformity is in the pelvic side.
- Total hip replacement remains the mainstay of treatment for advanced hip pathology.

Examination/Imaging

■ As part of the standard hip examination, range of motion, the presence of contractures, and leg length discrepancy should be assessed. The position of maximum comfort needs to be assessed in both sitting and standing positions and then correlated with the imaging findings.
■ Plain radiographs
  • Standing and supine anteroposterior (AP) pelvis and frog-leg lateral views should be obtained to evaluate the status of the hip joint with regard to the presence of osteoarthritis, femoral head subluxation, and the extent of femoral head involvement in the case of AVN.
  • Functional AP views in maximum hip abduction and adduction (which can also be done by fluoroscopy) are used to determine the range of motion of the hip joint and the presence of hinge abduction. The radiograph in Figure 9 of a

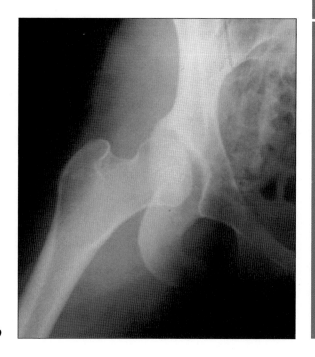

FIGURE 9

dysplastic hip in maximum abduction shows the femoral head fully contained.

- A false-profile pelvic view, which is a true lateral view of the hip joint, can provide good information such as anterior coverage of the femoral head in case of impingement or the extent of AVN in femoral head (Lequesne and De Seze, 1961).
- Preoperative planning is crucial for the success of a femoral osteotomy. Figure 10A shows the

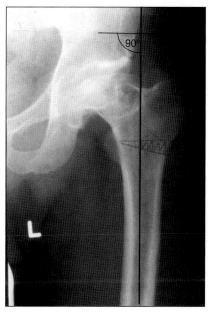
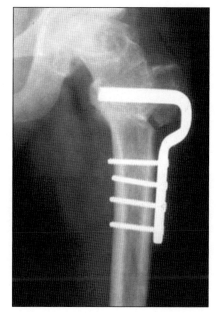

FIGURE 10   A   B

preoperative plan for a case of old Perthes disease. A valgus intertrochanteric osteotomy has been planned. Valgus correction was achieved and the osteotomy fixed with a 90° blade plate (Fig. 10B). In addition, the greater trochanter was transferred to improve the abductor lever arm.

- ◆ The level of resection and the amount of angular correction required should be decided on the basis of physical and radiologic examinations.
- ◆ The effect on leg length and the mechanical axis should also be anticipated.
- Magnetic resonance imaging
  - • In cases of AVN, it is helpful to assess the extent and site of the lesion in the femoral head before planning the osteotomy.
- Hip arthroscopy may be considered if there is a suspicion of a loose body or labral tear.

Surgical Anatomy

- In hip dysplasia, the femoral head is usually small, and the neck is excessively anteverted and possibly short. The neck-shaft angle is increased, and the greater trochanter is displaced posteriorly. On the pelvic side, the acetabulum is shallow and deficient superiorly and anteriorly, and tends to be anteverted (Sanchez-Sotelo et al., 2002).
- In slipped capital femoral epiphysis, the femoral head tends to be posterior, the neck is short, and the greater trochanter is overgrown.

Positioning

- The patient is positioned supine in a traction table without traction. The leg is draped completely free to allow manipulation.
- The contralateral leg needs to be positioned suitably to allow access of fluoroscopy equipment to obtain AP and lateral views of the hip.

Portals/Exposures

- A lateral incision is made extending 12 cm distally from the tip of greater trochanter.
- The vastus lateralis muscle split is performed close to the lateral intermuscular septum, and the muscle is retracted anteriorly (Fig. 11).

PITFALLS

- *Either the table wedge piece underneath the hip needs to be detached or a sandbag should be placed under the ischium to allow a better flexion-extension arc.*

Controversies

- This operation can be done when the patient is in a lateral decubitus position; however, access for the lateral fluoroscopic view will not be possible.

PITFALLS

- *If the vastus lateralis is lifted off the intermuscular septum, the bleeding perforators can be a nuisance to trace.*

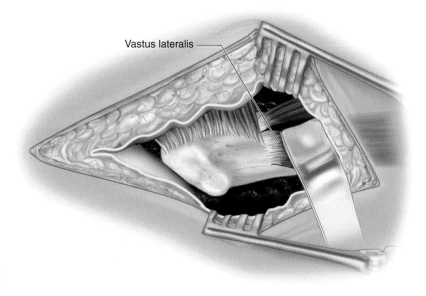

Vastus lateralis

FIGURE 11

Procedure

Step 1

■ A Kirschner wire (K-wire) is placed at the level of the lesser trochanter perpendicular to the shaft of the femur (Fig. 12). Fluoroscopy can be used at this stage to check the position of the lesser trochanter.

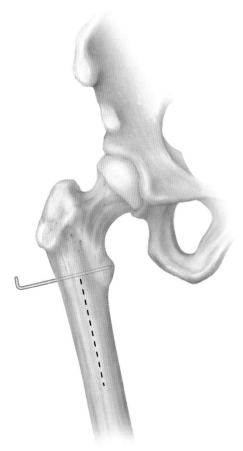

FIGURE 12

Instrumentation/ Implantation

- A blade plate with a 90° angle is commonly used for varus correction. Other implants, such as a dynamic condylar plate with a 95° angle, have also been used.
- For valgus osteotomy, a 120°-angle or 110°-angle blade plate is commonly used.

STEP 2

- A second K-wire is placed just proximal to the vastus lateralis ridge along the intended path of the blade. The position of this K-wire must be confirmed using fluoroscopy.
- The angle of this second K-wire relative to the first varies according to the desired angle of correction and the implant used to fix the osteotomy. For example:
  - If 20° of varus correction is desired, the second K-wire is placed at 20° from the first K-wire. The angle created with the femoral shaft will be 70° (Fig. 13A).
  - If 30° of valgus correction is desired, the second K-wire is placed parallel to the first K-wire at the intended path of the blade (Fig. 13B). Thus, when using a 120°-angle blade plate implant, the 30° valgus correction will be achieved when the plate is sitting on the femoral shaft (120 − 90 = 30).

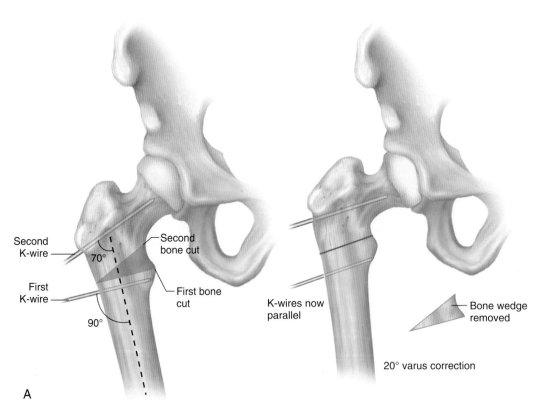

Second K-wire — 70°

Second bone cut

First K-wire

First bone cut

90°

K-wires now parallel

Bone wedge removed

20° varus correction

A

FIGURE 13

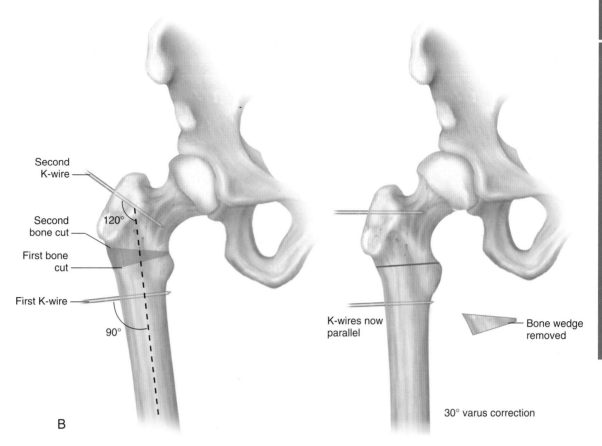

Second K-wire

Second bone cut

First bone cut

First K-wire

120°

90°

B

K-wires now parallel

Bone wedge removed

30° varus correction

FIGURE 13, cont'd

Step 3

■ The length of blade to be used is determined by measuring the length of the second K-wire in the bone with a depth gauge.

■ The chisel is inserted along the second K-wire. This should be done under fluoroscopic control until the final position of the blade is reached.

■ Rotation of the chisel should be checked carefully to allow the blade plate, when inserted, to sit on the lateral femur.

Step 4

■ Femoral osteotomy is done using a saw along the first K-wire. Continuous irrigation is required to avoid thermonecrosis.

■ If flexion or extension is contemplated, a small anterior or posterior wedge is cut, respectively.

Step 5

■ The proximal femur is displaced using a chisel and osteotome to achieve the planned correction. Using the saw, a small fragment from the medial cortex of the proximal segment is removed to achieve maximum contact at the osteotomy site. The proximal fragment is held with a bone reduction clamp.

Instrumentation/ Implantation

- A thin saw blade should be used to perform the osteotomy so as to avoid thermonecrosis.

- The chisel is removed and the blade plate is inserted under fluoroscopic control.
- One 4.5-mm screw is inserted in the proximal segment when the blade has reached its final seating.
- Using a bone clamp, the plate is seated on the femoral shaft and the rest of the screws are inserted.
- A final check is made with fluoroscopy. Hip range of motion is also checked.
- Figure 14 shows the repair of a dysplastic hip with a varus intertrochanteric osteotomy.
  - Preoperative planning was drawn on a radiograph of the left femur (Fig. 14A). Femoral head coverage was achieved in abduction, and the neck-shaft angle measured 150°. Therefore, 15° of correction was desirable.

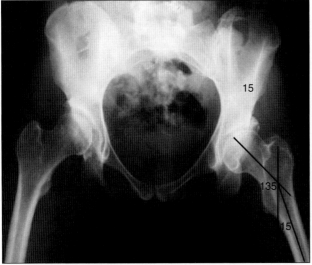

A

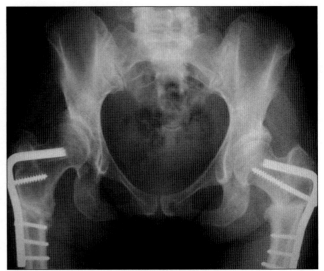

B

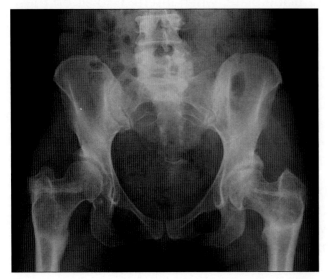

C

FIGURE 14

- The postoperative radiograph in Figure 14B shows that femoral head containment was achieved.
- Complete healing was achieved, and the metal implants were removed (Fig. 14C). Note that the intramedullary canal alignment is well maintained for future hip replacement.

PITFALLS

- *When displacing the proximal femoral segment, it must be kept in mind that the stem of a future total hip replacement needs to fit in the femoral canal. Therefore, minimal if any translation at the osteotomy site should be performed.*

- *Distraction at the osteotomy site should be avoided. Usually it tends to occur while performing varus osteotomy rather than with valgus osteotomy.*

Controversies

- Trendelenburg gait may persist following surgery, and distal transfer of the greater trochanter may be considered to address the abductor dysfunction.

Postoperative Care and Expected Outcomes

- The patient starts mobilization on the first postoperative day using crutches with toe-touch weight bearing for 6 weeks.
- In the second 6-week period, the patient starts gradually increasing weight bearing as tolerated. Continuous hip flexion and abduction exercises should also be performed during this period. Full weight bearing can be resumed more quickly following valgus osteotomy.
- Removal of the blade plate after 18 months is controversial but routinely done in many institutions.
- The possible complications, such as intraoperative fracture, loss of fixation, and nonunion, are fairly uncommon (Iwase et al., 1996). The patient should be warned about postoperative leg length discrepancy, and the persistence or worsening of the lurch.
- Overall, the results of femoral osteotomy in well-selected patients with minimal hip arthritic changes are satisfactory. Studies have shown that over 70% of patients have had a satisfactory result following varus osteotomy (Iwase et al., 1996; Pellicci et al., 1991).
- The results of valgus osteotomy can be less predictable or at least not as successful as varus osteotomy. Studies have shown that less than 50% and 40% of patients were satisfied with the results of

valgus osteotomy for hip dysplasia and idiopathic osteoarthritis, respectively (Perlau et al., 1996). However, valgus osteotomy for femoral neck fracture nonunion gives excellent results in achieving fracture union (Marti et al., 1989).

Evidence

D'Souza SR, Sadiq S, New AM, Northmore-Ball MD. Proximal femoral osteotomy as the primary operation for young adults who have osteoarthrosis of the hip. J Bone Joint Surg Am. 1998;80:1428–38.

A retrospective study of 25 hips in 23 patients with an average follow-up of 7 years. (Level III evidence)

Iwase T, Hasegawa Y, Kawamoto K, Iwasada S, Yamada K, Iwata H. Twenty years' followup of intertrochanteric osteotomy for treatment of the dysplastic hip. Clin Orthop Relat Res. 1996;(331):245–55.

A cohort study of 110 hips in 95 patients over a mean follow-up of 20 years. (Level III evidence)

Lequesne M, De Seze S. False profile of the pelvis: a new radiographic incidence for the study of the hip. Its use in dysplasias and different coxopathies. Rev Rhum Mal Osteoartic. 1961;28:643–52.

Marti RK, Schuller HM, Raaymakers EL. Intertrochanteric osteotomy for non-union of the femoral neck. J Bone Joint Surg Br. 1989;71:782–7.

A cohort study of 50 patients over an average follow-up of 7.1 years. (Level III evidence)

Pellicci PM, Hu S, Garvin KL, Salvati EA, Wilson PD Jr. Varus rotational femoral osteotomies in adults with hip dysplasia. Clin Orthop. 1991;(272):162–6.

A cohort study of 56 hips in 48 patients over a mean follow-up of 12.5 years. (Level III evidence)

Perlau R, Wilson MG, Poss R. Isolated proximal femoral osteotomy for treatment of residua of congenital dysplasia or idiopathic osteoarthrosis of the hip: five to ten-year results. J Bone Joint Surg Am. 1996;78:1462–7.

A retrospective study of 34 hips in 33 patients over a mean follow-up of 6.1 years. (Level III evidence)

Sanchez-Sotelo J, Berry DJ, Trousdale RT, Cabanela ME. Surgical treatment of developmental dysplasia of the hip in adults: I. Nonarthroplasty options. J Am Acad Orthop Surg. 2002;10:321–33.

A review of non-joint replacement treatment of mild to moderate symptomatic hip dysplasia in young adults. (Level IV evidence [review article])

Santore RF, Turgeon TR, Phillips WF 3rd, Kantor SR. Pelvic and femoral osteotomy in the treatment of hip disease in the young adult. Instr Course Lect. 2006;55:131–44.

A review article detailing the authors extensive experience in the treatment of mild to moderate hip arthritis by means of both femoral and pelvic osteotomy with detailed results. (Level IV evidence [review article])

Bernese Periacetabular Osteotomy

Michael B. Millis

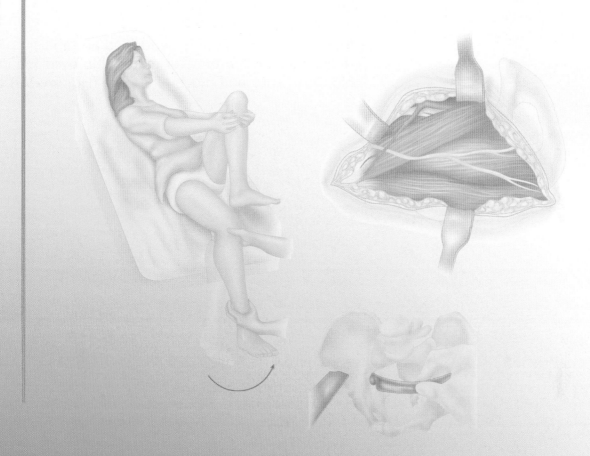

PITFALLS

- *Open triradiate cartilage (posterior column portion of osteotomy would disrupt remaining growth)*

- *Femoroacetabular incongruity*

- *Severe osteoarthrosis*

Controversies

- Borderline indications include the older patient with moderate osteoarthrosis, for whom replacement arthroplasty is an option.

Introduction

- The Bernese periacetabular osteotomy is a powerful acetabular redirection procedure performed by making a series of connecting cuts to free up the acetabulum without disturbing the posterior column.

- It can be performed without abductor dissection, and it can easily be combined with an anterior arthrotomy for intra-articular surgery. Stable fixation allows early postoperative ambulation.

- It is the most commonly performed acetabular redirectional osteotomy for mature hip dysplasia in North America and much of Europe (Fig. 1A–1D).

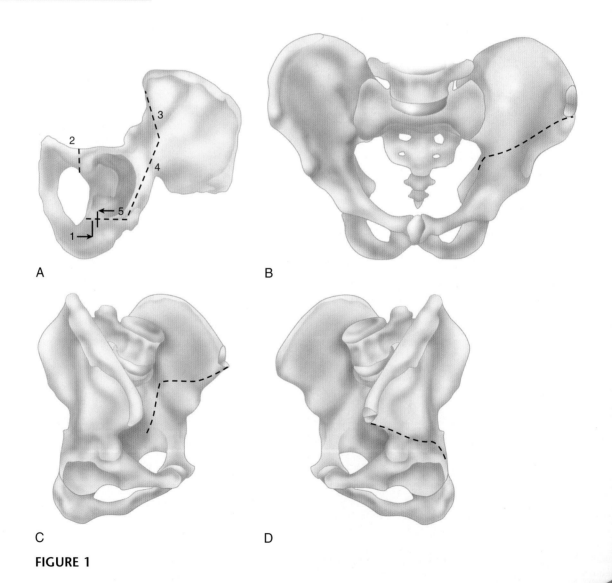

A

B

C

D

FIGURE 1

Indications

- Symptomatic congruous acetabular dysplasia in a skeletally mature patient with zero to mild osteoarthrosis

Examination/Imaging

PHYSICAL EXAMINATION

- Range of motion (ROM)
  - Passive ROM—flex and extend hip.
  - Limited range implies arthrosis.
- Anterior impingement test
  - Hip flexion, adduction, and internal rotation produces groin pain secondary to anterior acetabular pathology (Fig. 2).
  - Positive test implies damage to rim tissues. *Not* specific for labral tear.

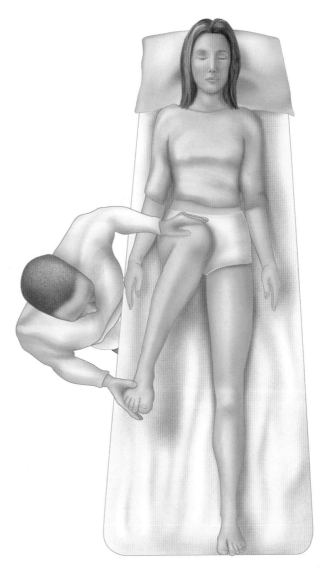

FIGURE 2

Treatment Options

- *Joint-preserving options:* Proximal femoral redirection osteotomy may be an alternative in cases in which both mild acetabular dysplasia and mild to moderate proximal femoral deformity are present. In general, in cases in which mild to moderate deformity is present at both the acetabular and femoral levels,

- Apprehension test
  - Anterior instability is shown by hip extension, adduction, and external rotation producing discomfort secondary to deficient anterior acetabular coverage (Fig. 3).
  - Positive test suggests anterior instability. Commonly positive in acetabular dysplasia.
- Bicycle test
  - Repetitive cycles, especially against resistance at the foot, will produce pain secondary to abductor fatigue. Abductor musculature is palpated for tenderness (Fig. 4).
  - Positive test suggests abductor overload. Commonly positive in acetabular dysplasia.

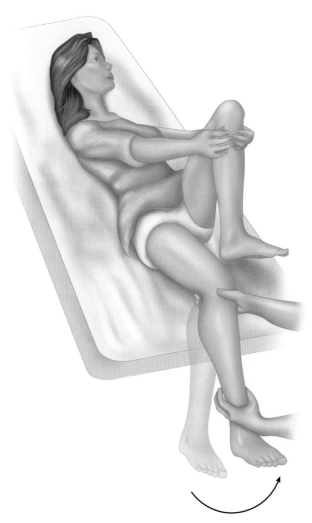

FIGURE 3

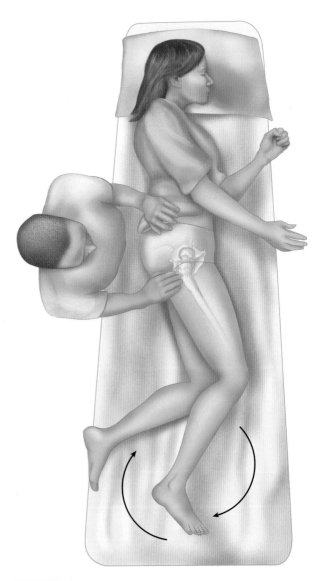

FIGURE 4

Treatment Options —cont'd

acetabular redirection to achieve a physiologic acetabular alignment is more likely to achieve satisfying clinical results than is a femoral osteotomy, which leaves acetabular deformity uncorrected.

- *Chiari pelvic osteotomy:* Chiari osteotomy is a stabilizing procedure that utilizes an iliac shelf to buttress the capsule, providing stability but not support for the femoral head by true hyaline cartilage. Chiari osteotomy is useful in moderately incongruous dysplastic hips but does not provide a physiologic reconstruction likely to provide long-term function as satisfactory as rotation of hyaline acetabular cartilage over the femoral head.
- *Total hip replacement arthroplasty:* This is a reasonable alternative to periacetabular osteotomy if the patient is relatively old and the arthrosis in the hip is moderately advanced.

PLAIN RADIOGRAPHS

- Standing anteroposterior radiograph of the pelvis centered on the femoral heads is standard (Fig. 5A).
  - Femoroacetabular congruity can be assessed, as can be the amount of dysplasia, as measured by the lateral center-edge angle and the tilt of the weight-bearing zone (Tönnis angle). Most symptomatic dysplastic hips have a lateral center-edge angle of less than 15° (lower limit of normal is about 25°). Upper limit of normal for roof angle tilt is about 10°; most symptomatic dysplastic hips have a roof angle tilt of more than 15°.
  - Version of the acetabulum can be roughly assessed by the point at which the anterior and posterior rims meet, with their convergence in a point at the lateral edge of the weight-bearing zone reflecting a normally anteverted acetabulum. Crossing over of the anterior and posterior rims more medially suggests acetabular retroversion.
- False-profile view, which is a 65° lateral standing view, is a sagittal view of the acetabulum, demonstrating anterior coverage of the femoral head by the acetabulum. The lower limit of the anterior center-edge angle is 20° (Fig. 5B).
- Von Rosen view (flexion-abduction–internal rotation, taken supine).
  - An optional, functional radiograph to simulate coverage by either acetabular or femoral redirection.
  - Useful if passive hip motion is limited and incongruity or hinging is suspected.

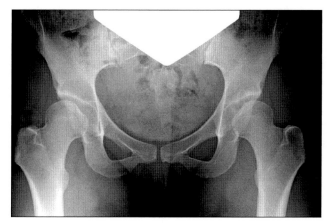 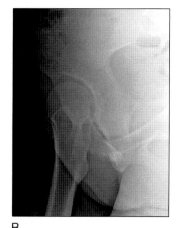

FIGURE 5 A   B

- Most useful with gadolinium contrast.
- Directly demonstrates both the labrum and the articular cartilage. Useful in assessing labral pathology and character of the acetabular cartilage, which can be very useful in the borderline hip with some arthrosis, since in dysplasia, severe cartilage damage can have occurred at a stage at which the thickness of the cartilage is not yet compromised (Fig. 6).

Surgical Anatomy

- Detailed knowledge of the soft tissue and bony anatomy encountered during the anterior Smith-Petersen approach to the hip is essential (Fig. 7). The lateral femoral cutaneous nerve crosses the interval between the sartorius and tensor and must be carefully protected as it is carried medially when the supra-acetabular ilium and capsule are exposed.
- The femoral neurovascular structures lie anterior and medial to the psoas tendon and are well protected if the continuity of the psoas tendon is respected and the hip is flexed and adducted during dissection anterior and medial to the hip joint.
- The sciatic nerve exits the pelvis through the greater sciatic notch and courses distal to the sciatic notch posterior and lateral to the hip joint. It is protected both by avoiding dissection within the sciatic notch itself and by maintaining the hip relatively extended and abducted when the portions of the osteotomy are made along the posterior column and across the ischium.

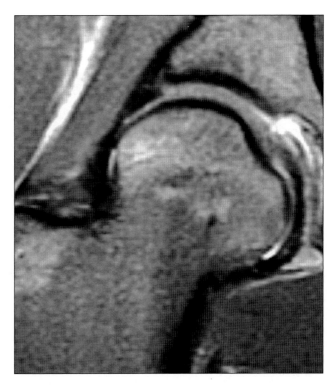

FIGURE 6

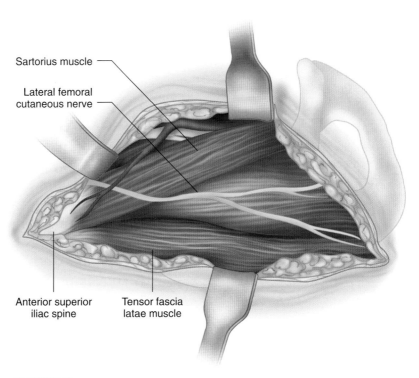

Sartorius muscle

Lateral femoral
cutaneous nerve

Anterior superior
iliac spine

Tensor fascia
latae muscle

FIGURE 7

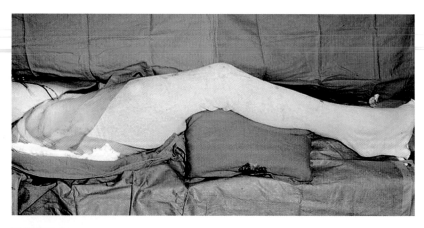

FIGURE 8

Equipment

• Positioning equipment: image intensification control during the case is highly useful, especially for the less experienced surgeon.

Positioning

■ The patient is positioned supine on a radiolucent table. The routine approach for Bernese periacetabular osteotomy is anterior. The optimal exposure for the experienced surgeon involves the medial half of the Smith-Petersen approach, the so-called direct anterior approach.

■ The ipsilateral lower extremity and flank are prepped and draped, with the extremity free (Fig. 8). The proximal limit of the sterile field is the costal margin. The medial aspect of the prepped area is the midline down to the groin. Laterally, the sterile field reaches posteriorly to the midbuttock.

Portals/Exposures

■ The Smith-Petersen exposure can be made through either of two incisions. The most user-friendly incision for the surgeon is a longitudinal incision convex medially, centered just distal and lateral to the anterior superior spine (Fig. 9A). An alternative incision, which is more cosmetic but less useful in achieving extensive visualization distally and medially, is convex proximal-medially, and centered just distal to the anterior superior spine.

■ Dissection into the Smith-Petersen interval between the sartorius and tensor precedes osteotomy of a small block of bone from the anterior superior spine, which releases the sartorius and inguinal ligament and the inguinal ligament insertion to allow more extensive exposure of the capsule and superior ramus without excessive tension on soft tissues medially (Fig. 9B).

Instrumentation

• If direct visualization of all portions of the osteotomy is required, then the ilioinguinal approach, utilizing an additional window medial to the psoas, is required. This is rarely if ever necessary unless complex post-traumatic deformity is encountered.

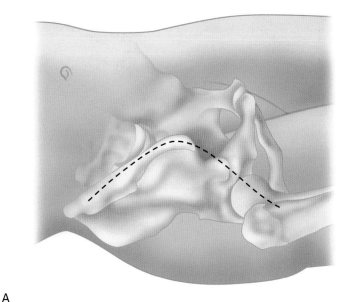

A

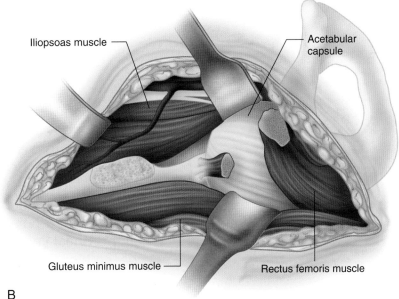

Iliopsoas muscle — Acetabular capsule

Gluteus minimus muscle — Rectus femoris muscle

B

FIGURE 9

■ If arthrotomy is to be performed to examine the rim and labrum, and to carry out neck osteoplasty, the straight head of the rectus and the iliocapsularis are dissected sharply off the capsule in a distal and medial direction, facilitated by flexing and adducting the hip.

■ The medial half of the iliac crest is exposed subperiosteally without disturbing the abductors. Flexing and adducting the hip allows the medial wall of the ilium to be subperiosteally exposed to and below the iliopectineal line into the true pelvis.

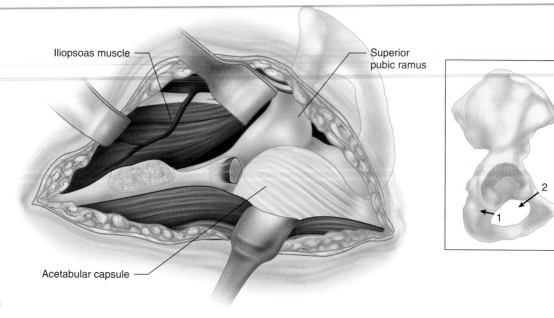

Iliopsoas muscle

Superior
pubic ramus

Acetabular capsule

FIGURE 10

Controversies

• If direct visualization of all
portions of the osteotomy are
required, then the ilioinguinal
approach, utilizing an additional
window medial to the psoas is
required. This is rarely if ever
necessary unless complex
posttraumatic deformity is
encountered.

PEARLS

• *Initial blunt enlarging of the
interval between the psoas
tendon and the capsule is useful
to allow the forked chisel to be
passed safely until its tip lies on
the bone of the ischium just
below the acetabulum.*

• *Image intensifier control is useful
to confirm that the direction of
the osteotomy is roughly parallel
to the inferior acetabulum (see
Fig. 11B and 11C). It should not
be directed too distally.*

PITFALLS

• *With the hip moderately flexed,
as it must be for the chisel to be
passed onto the groove safely, the
sciatic nerve lies just lateral to
the ischium. The osteotomy must
not be directed laterally to avoid
injury to the sciatic nerve.*

■ The superior pubic ramus is exposed subperiosteally
to a point at least 1 cm medial to the iliopectineal
eminence, remaining deep to the psoas tendon and
femoral neurovascular structures. This is facilitated by
flexing and adducting the hip (Fig. 10).

■ The posterior column and medial ischium are
exposed to a point at least 5 cm below the
iliopectineal line, facilitated by flexion and adduction
of the hip. Dissection into the sciatic notch is
avoided. A reverse Hohmann retractor placed on the
ischial spine facilitates exposure of the medial
ischium and the lateral edge of the obturator
foramen.

■ The obturator membrane is elevated from the
superolateral corner of the obturator foramen both
inside and outside the pelvis.

■ The infracotyloid groove of the ischium is dissected
subperiosteally by passing a blunt retractor into the
interval anteriorly between the medial hip joint
capsule and the psoas tendon. Image intensifier
control is useful in placing this dissection directly in
the groove in which runs the obturator externus
tendon. The dissection must be distal to the inferior
lip of the acetabulum yet proximal to the obturator
externus tendon, which itself lies just proximal to the
important medial femoral circumflex artery.

Procedure

STEP 1: OSTEOTOMY CUT 1

- The ischial osteotomy is performed with an angled forked Synthes chisel impacted into the infracotyloid groove of the ischium just inferior to the hip joint capsule but proximal to the obturator externus tendon (Fig. 11A–11C; see also Fig. 1).

Instrumentation/Implantation

- Use of a forked angled chisel, such as the Ganz osteotomes, is recommended for the ischial osteotomy, since its forked shape allows good control of the instrument as the strong ischial bone is cut.

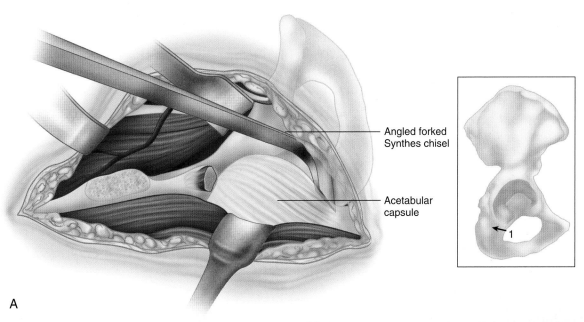

Angled forked Synthes chisel

Acetabular capsule

A

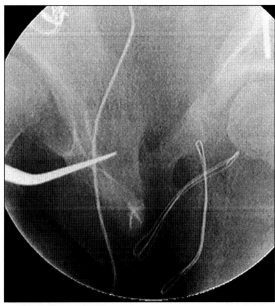

B

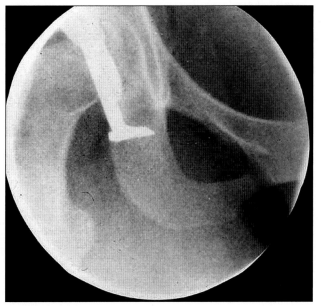

C

FIGURE 11

Controversies

- Extending the ischial osteotomy posteriorly along the medial wall of the ilium is an option that sometimes facilitates final freeing up of the fragment later in the operation. If done, it is done with an angled chisel introduced inside the pelvis, lateral to the iliacus, with the tip of the angled chisel placed against the medial wall at least 4 cm below the iliopectineal line. Image intensifier control in an oblique projection is useful to confirm that this cut is placed about 1 cm below the joint, which is ideal. The chisel can be advanced stepwise posteriorly, after cuts are made through the medial cortex and to but not through the lateral cortex. This stepwise posterior extension of the ischial osteotomy can be continued until the posterior column is reached, just superficial to the ischial spine and about 1 cm anterior to the anterior edge of the greater sciatic notch.

PEARLS

- *This osteotomy is directed from anteriorly and laterally to posteriorly and medially, perpendicular to the long axis of the superior ramus. This direction minimizes the risk of joint penetration and facilitates displacement of the superior ramus osteotomy during fragment reorientation.*

- *Extensive blunt dissection of the obturator membrane away from the supralateral obturator foramen both anteriorly and posteriorly facilitates placement of retractors under the ramus to protect the obturator nerve and vessels.*

- *The Gigli saw may be passed with a suture under the ramus to allow an osteotomy to be made in a deep to superficial direction, which minimizes risk to obturator neurovascular structures and guarantees completeness of the osteotomy.*

- *If radiographic control is necessary, a Kirschner wire marking the site of the proposed osteotomy should lie medial to the teardrop.*

- The chisel is inserted into the interval between the psoas tendon and the hip joint capsule, with the hip flexed and adducted.
- The chisel is directed from anterior to posterior, maintaining a bridge below the hip joint of at least 5–7 mm.
- The chisel is impacted to a depth of about 2 cm.

STEP 2: OSTEOTOMY CUT 2

- The second cut divides the superior pubic ramus, just medial to the iliopectineal eminence (Fig. 12A and 12B). Either a straight chisel or a Gigli saw is employed.

- *Neurovascular structures both deep and superficial to the superior ramus must be carefully protected during the osteotomy. Hip flexion and adduction is useful.*

Instrumentation/ Implantation

- Blunt Hohmann retractors or Rang retractors are useful for exposure of the superior pubic ramus and protection of the obturator structures.

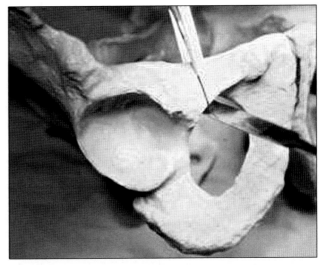

A

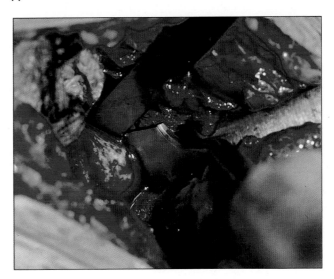

B

FIGURE 12

STEP 3: OSTEOTOMY CUT 3

- The third cut is that of the ilium proximal to the acetabulum (Fig. 13A–13C).
- It is made with an oscillating saw in an anteroposterior direction, which is vertical in attitude as the patient lies in a supine position. The cut is made with adequate protection of the soft tissues on both the medial and lateral sides of the ilium.
- The saw cut begins just distal to the anterior superior spine and is directed vertically in the direction of the apex of the sciatic notch. The abductor origin is not disturbed. The cut stops about 1 cm short of the iliopectineal line.

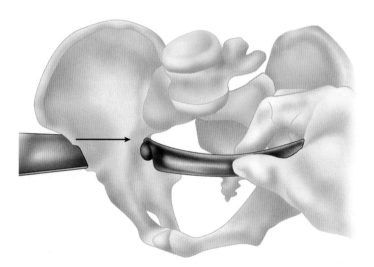

A

FIGURE 13

Controversies

- If the anatomy is unusual or the surgeon's experience with this procedure is limited, then reflexion of the abductor muscles off the lateral wall of the ilium, as in the classic Smith-Petersen exposure, can confirm directly the appropriate attitude of the saw cut. This increases the risk of abductor dysfunction following the procedure but may reduce the risk of direct injury to the abductor muscles that inexperience may cause.

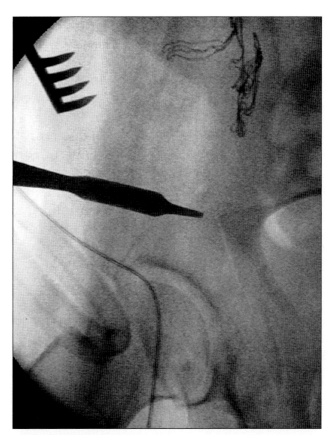

B

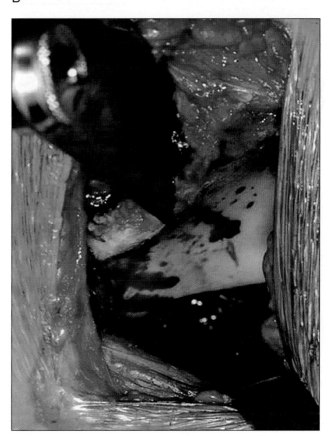

C

FIGURE 13, cont'd

PEARLS

- *Image intensifier control is useful to confirm that the chisel is remaining anterior to and parallel to the anterior edge of the sciatic notch and posterior to the posterior edge of the acetabulum. Ideally this cut bisects the posterior column (Fig. 14B).*

- *This cut continues in a deep direction toward the ischial spine until it is at least 4 cm below the iliopectineal line.*

- *Angling the chisel so that its lateral edge is slightly posterior to its medial edge facilitates the chisel's passing into the thinner bone closer to the sciatic notch and directs the chisel away from the acetabulum, as desired.*

- *At its deepest extent, the posterior column osteotomy should be angled slightly anteriorly, to be directed somewhat toward the previously made osteotomy.*

STEP 4: OSTEOTOMY CUT 4 (POSTERIOR COLUMN OSTEOTOMY)

- The posterior column osteotomy begins at the posterior end of the saw cut, just superficial to the iliopectineal line (Fig. 14A).
- It is made with a straight osteotome, passes over the iliopectineal line, and is directed at the ischial spine.
- This cut is made along the medial wall of the ilium and initially goes to, but not completely through, the lateral cortex of the posterior column. It splits the posterior column, remaining parallel to and about 1 cm anterior to the anterior edge of the sciatic notch.

PITFALLS

- *Angling the osteotomy either toward the sciatic notch or toward the joint is to be avoided.*

- *The sciatic nerve is in close proximity to this posterior column osteotomy. The hip should therefore be nearly fully extended and abducted, and the knee flexed slightly to relax the sciatic nerve while the posterior column osteotomy is being performed.*

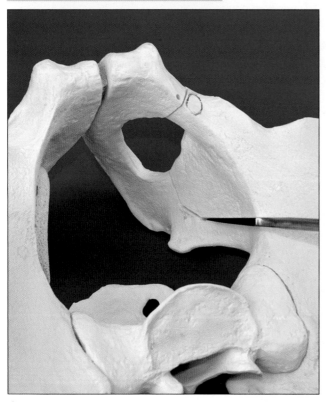

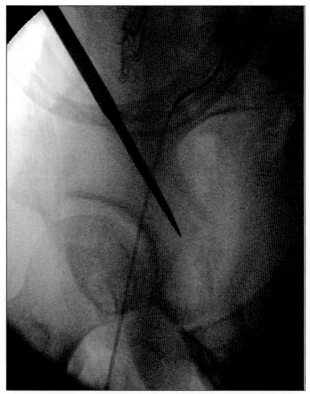

A

B

FIGURE 14

STEP 5: OSTEOTOMY CUT 5 (POSTERIOR ISCHIAL OSTEOTOMY)

- The remaining osteotomy involves direct cutting or indirect fracture of the small remaining bridge of ischial bone under the acetabulum (Fig. 15A–15C).

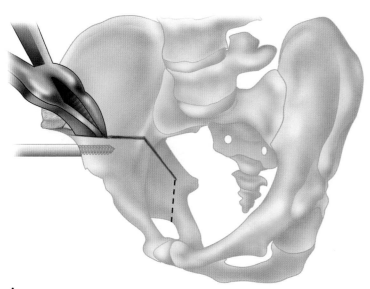

A

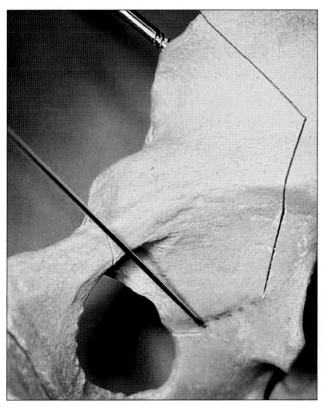

B

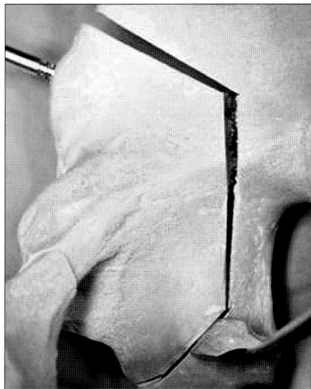

C

FIGURE 15

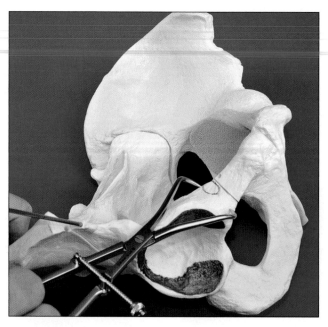

FIGURE 16

- Placement of a Schanz screw from anterior to posterior in the acetabular fragment allows the fragment to be extended to stress this small remaining bridge of bone. Simultaneous placement of a bone spreader in the anterior portion of the iliac osteotomy allows further stressing of the intact bony bridge.

- The fragment is thus extended and everted, and internal torque applied through the Schanz screw usually will fracture the remaining deep bone bridges, completing the periacetabular osteotomy.

STEP 6: ACETABULAR FRAGMENT MOBILIZATION AND REORIENTATION

- Since the usual dysplastic acetabulum is insufficient both anteriorly and laterally, rotating the fragment mostly in the anterior direction is appropriate; this tends to give some lateral coverage as well. This is performed by pulling anteriorly and inferiorly with the Schanz screw to rotate the fragment in place. Slight internal rotation of the fragment as it is rotated anteriorly helps to avoid undesired retroversion (Fig. 17A–17C).

- Provisional fixation of the fragment in a corrected position is achieved with smooth Kirschner wires through the iliac crest into the extra-articular portions of the acetabular fragment; 3/32-inch smooth Kirschner wires are useful (Fig. 17D).

- Imaging is carried out to confirm that the desired horizontalization of the weight-bearing zone of the

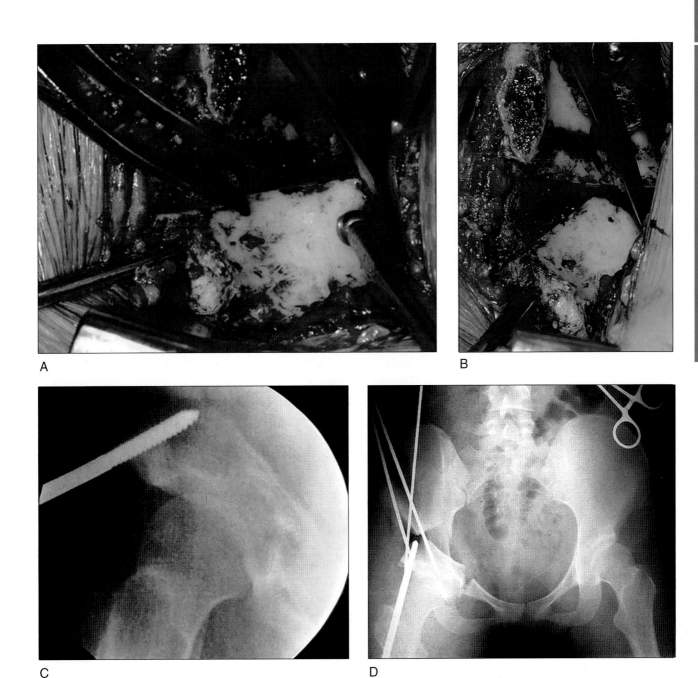

A

B

C

D

FIGURE 17

acetabulum has been achieved, that retroversion has been avoided, and that lateralization also has been avoided. Shenton's line should be restored and congruence maintained.

- Passive hip flexion and abduction is checked; 90° of passive hip flexion should be maintained. Direct palpation over the anterior capsule should be carried out as the hip is flexed. If any suggestion of impingement is present, then anterior arthrotomy should be carried out and either reduction and correction considered or osteoplasty of the femoral neck to increase offset considered.

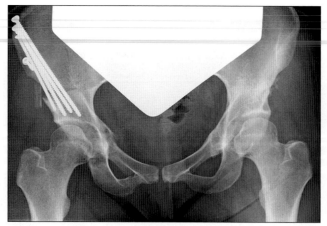 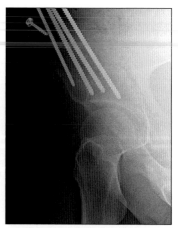

A   B

FIGURE 18

- Definitive fixation is achieved by multiple long cortical screws drilled through the iliac crest into the extra-articular portions of the acetabular fragment. Three or four 4.5-mm screws are usually sufficient. Supplementation of the fixation with an anterior-to-posterior, so-called home run screw from the anterior inferior spine area into the posterior column above the sciatic notch may be useful (Fig. 18A and 18B).
- Trimming of jagged edges, particularly at the superior ramus level and at the anterior inferior spine level, is useful, with this bone being used to pack into the osteotomy clefts.

STEP 7: ANTERIOR ARTHROTOMY

- Anterior arthrotomy is carried out in most cases, both to confirm that no unstable labral tear is present and to confirm that no femoroacetabular impingement has been created by the acetabular correction.
- A T-shaped anterior capsulotomy is easy to perform and involves no risk to the blood supply to the femoral head (Fig. 19).
- The labrum is examined and débrided if an unstable tear is present. The hip is carefully flexed, abducted, and internally rotated with the capsule open, and any potential impingement is eliminated, either by reducing the amount of acetabular redirection as mentioned above, or by anterolateral femoral neck osteoplasty, or by a combination.
- The capsule is then loosely closed after hemostasis of any area of bone resection is achieved.

STEP 8: SOFT TISSUE REPAIR

- Soft tissue repair routinely is carried out with absorbable suture.

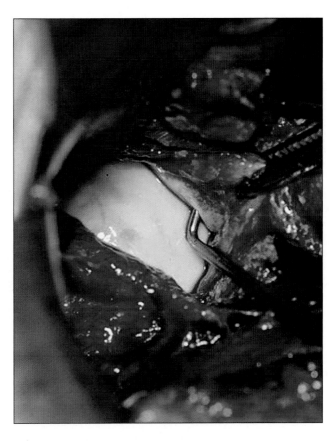

FIGURE 19

- If the rectus has been dissected, it is repaired through a drill hole through bone.
- The medial iliac periosteum is sutured to the ilium through drill holes.
- The anterior superior spine osteotomy is anatomically repaired with a 4.0-mm cancellous screw and washer (Fig. 20).

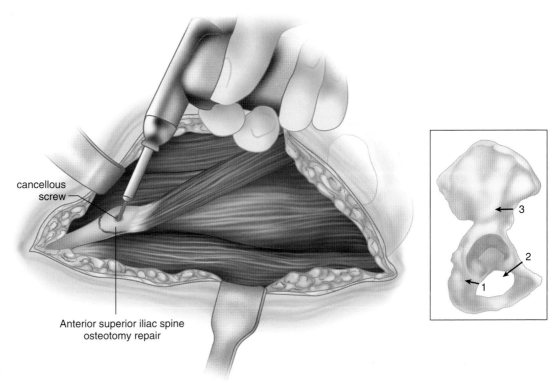

cancellous screw

Anterior superior iliac spine osteotomy repair

FIGURE 20

Postoperative Care and Expected Outcomes

- Endotracheal anesthesia with continuous epidural supplementation is routine. Continous epidural anesthesia routinely is employed for 48–72 hours postoperatively, with general ROM active assisted exercises carried out even while in bed. A continuous passive motion machine is employed if extensive intra-articular work has been done.
- Mobilization to a partial weight-bearing gait with two crutches begins on the third postoperative day.
- Antigravity exercises are avoided until good leg control and bony healing are seen, usually at 6–8 weeks following surgery.
- Postoperative anticoagulation is used in adult patients.

Evidence

Ganz R, Klaue K, Vinh TS, Mast JW. A new periacetabular osteotomy for the treatment of hip dysplasia. Clin Orthop. 1988;232:26–36.

This is the classical original description of Bernese periacetabular osteotomy, including the original series from Berne. (Level IV evidence)

Harris WH. Etiology of osteoarthritis of the hip. Clin Orthop. 1986;213:20–33.

Dr. Harris' interesting essay elucidates his thesis that nearly all, or perhaps all osteoarthritis of the hip is secondary. He suggests developmental abnormalities and deformities as the commonest etiologic factors in the development of OA in the hip. (Level V evidence)

Kim YJ, Jaramillo D, Millis MB, Gray M, Burstein D. Assessment of early osteoarthritis in hip dysplasia with delayed gadolinium-enhanced magnetic resonance imaging of cartilage. J Bone Joint Surg Am. 2003;85A:1987–92.

Kim et al present an innovative and potentially extremely useful non-invasive imaging technique for assessing the functional integrity of articular cartilage in the mature dysplastic hip. This so-called dGEMRIC technique correlated much better with symptoms than either plain radiographic measures or more standard MR. (Level III evidence)

Leunig M, Siebenrock KA, Ganz R. Rationale of periacetabular osteotomy and background work. Instr Course Lect. 2001;50:229–38.

This is an in-depth analysis of the mechanical and clinical rationale for periacetabular osteotomy, presented in clear fashion by the originator of the technique and co-workers. (Level V evidence)

Millis MB, Murphy SB. [The Boston concept. Peri-acetabular osteotomy with simultaneous arthrotomy via direct anterior approach]. Orthopade. 1998;27:751–8.

This series of periacetabular osteotomies carried out with simultaneous anterior arthrotomy documents the relatively high frequency of labral tears in symptomatic dysplastic hips treated by periacetabular osteotomy, ranging from more than 20% in hips treated during the third decade to more than 40% in hips treated during the fifth decade of life. (Level IV evidence)

Millis MB. Reconstructive osteotomies of the pelvis for the correction of acetabular dysplasia. In Sledge CB (ed). Master Techniques in Orthopaedic Surgery. New York: Lippincott-Raven, 1998:157–82.

This well-illustrated chapter outlines well both indications and techniques of rotational acetabular osteotomy and Bernese periacetabular osteotomy. The descriptions are somewhat dated in that the emphasis is given to the classic Smith-Petersen exposure of both inner and outer wall of the pelvic, rather than the more contemporary abductor-sparing exposures. (Level V evidence)

Millis MB, Kim YJ. Rationale of osteotomy and related procedures for hip preservation: a review. Clin Orthop. 2002;405:108–21.

This broad-based review presents the contemporary mechanistic paradigm for the prevention and treatment of osteoarthrosis in the hip by realignment osteotomy. (Level V evidence)

Millis MB, Murphy SB. Periacetabular osteotomy. In Callaghan J, Rosenberg AG, Rubash HE (eds). The Adult Hip. Philadelphia: Lippincott Williams & Wilkins, 2007:795–815.

This is a contemporary complete presentation of the indications for, the use of, and the relevant techniques involved in periacetabular osteotomy. (Level V evidence)

Murphy SB, Millis MB. Periacetabular osteotomy without abductor dissection using direct anterior exposure. Clin Orthop. 1999;364:92–8.

This important study describes the now-standard abductor-sparing approach for periacetabular osteotomy, emphasizing the possibility for the osteotomy to be carried out by the experienced surgeon without disrupting the abductor origin. (Level V evidence)

Murphy SB, Deshmukh R. Periacetabular osteotomy: preoperative radiographic predictors of outcome. Clin Orthop. 2002;405:168–74.

Murphy and Deshmukh document the importance of punctual radiographs in determining likely outcome of periacetabular osteotomy. Hinging detected on functional radiographs predicted high risk of poor outcome. (Level IV evidence)

PRIMARY TOTAL HIP ARTHROPLASTY

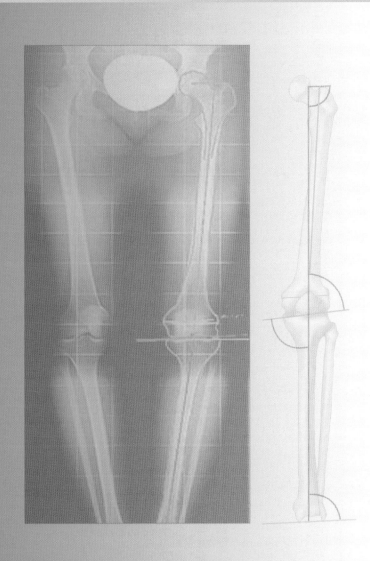

Templating for Primary Total Hip Arthroplasty

Mahmoud A. Hafez and Emil H. Schemitsch

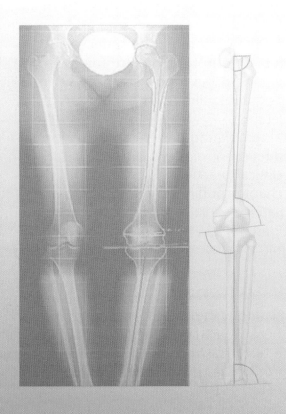

Introduction

- Templating is a familiar terminology to orthopedic surgeons whether it is used preoperatively or intraoperatively.
    - Templating has been extensively used for preoperative planning of fracture fixation and total joint arthroplasty.
    - Intraoperative templates have been routinely used to know the size and the shape of metallic plates before the latter are selected and contoured to fit the corresponding bone surfaces.
    - Templating in total hip arthroplasty (THA) is not new, and it has long been used with traditional radiographic films and printed templates (acetates).
- Digital templating has become possible with the introduction of digital radiography and computers into clinical practice.
- This chapter outlines the indications and rationale for templating, explains different methods used, and then describes in more detail the technical steps and possible pitfalls.

Indications

- Templating is indicated for every primary THA whether it is a straightforward or a complicated case.
    - The technical success of THA requires accurate and reproducible preoperative planning (Knight and Atwater, 1992).
    - Prevention of complications such as dislocation and leg length inequality is dependent on the precision of alignment and position of prosthetic components (Morrey, 1992).
    - The hip joint is deep and, even with maximum exposure, many of the anatomic details and landmarks are not visible.
    - The introduction of limited and minimally invasive techniques for THA has increased the demand for accurate and reliable preoperative planning.
- Templating can help in deciding the type of fixation needed, whether cemented, cementless, or hybrid.
    - Bone stock is important, and it is useful to know in advance the cup size and the level of femoral neck cut to facilitate minimal bone removal.
    - Center of rotation has to be restored, offset needs to be optimized, and alignment of the stem should be anatomic.

PEARLS

- *Benefits of templating include*

- *Identification of difficult or problematic cases such as narrow femoral canals that require smaller stems than what are available*

- *Accurate documentation of preoperative leg length discrepancy*

- *Planning for leg length equalization and estimating the level of the femoral neck cut*

- *Restoration of the normal hip center*

- *Optimization of femoral offset*

- *Prediction of sizes of femoral and acetabular implants*

- *Making surgeons more familiar with the normal and abnormal anatomy of the hip joint*

- *Training tool for junior surgeons*

- Leg length, ideally, should be equal particularly after the increasing rate of litigation in North America due to leg length discrepancy.
- Templating alerts the surgeon to otherwise unexpected intraoperative difficulties and complications.
  - Surgeons should be aware well in advance regarding unusual implants or instruments. Larger femoral heads or constrained cups may be required if a higher risk of dislocation is expected.
  - The difficulty related to keeping a complete inventory of implants and instrumentation is another concern. In smaller institutions or centers where the turnover of THA cases is not large, manufacturers may supply a limited stock of implants. In such cases, templating is useful in predicting implant sizes and in providing adequate inventory.
- Several authors have found that preoperative planning is useful in predicting implant size, position, and alignment, as well as in restoring the center of rotation, and equalizing limb length (Bono, 2004; Carter et al., 1995; Davila et al., 2006; Della Valle et al., 2005).
- The accuracy of templating increases gradually with the level of training (Carter et al. 1995).

Materials and Methods

- Radiographs should include an anteroposterior (AP) view of the pelvis (both hips) and both AP and lateral views of the affected hip that include the acetabulum and the proximal third of the femur.
  - Patient positioning is critical to avoid misleading information.
  - The x-ray magnification has to be taken into account and be corrected before templating is started (Conn et al., 2002).
  - Templating can be done whether using printed acetates or specific software. The printed acetates may be applied to radiographic films or digital images.
- Radiographic films are still frequently used in many hospitals around the world, but the use of digital imaging is on the rise.
  - In the United States, it has been estimated that 60% of hospitals have digital imaging (filmless). Digital images allow the use of powerful software

with better functionality and more accurate measurements (Murzic et al., 2005).

TRADITIONAL TEMPLATING

- In this method, surgeons lay and match printed acetates (templates) of implants over radiographic films. The acetates are usually magnified to a certain number of degrees to compensate for x-ray magnification. Manufacturers usually provide information about the percentage of magnification of the templates.

TEMPLATING WITH ACETATES OVER DIGITAL IMAGES

- This technique involves the use of printed acetates with digital images rather than radiographic films. The technique has been found to be accurate and reproducible (Oddy et al., 2006), but White and Shardlow (2005) found digital images could reduce the magnification of the film and, therefore, reduce the accuracy of preoperative templates supplied by the manufacturers of implants, resulting in incorrect selection of implant.

DIGITAL TEMPLATING

- In this method, the templating is entirely performed using specific software. There is automatic scaling once the degree of magnification is selected, thus correcting the magnification on the displayed radiographic images.
- The software has a library of implants from different manufacturers in various sizes, which can be imported and superimposed on the radiographic images in coronal or sagittal views. The implants can be manipulated by translation or angulation until the optimal position is achieved. Measurements of leg length, distances, and angles can be done in decimals.
- Several software systems are available, such as OrthoView, OrthWork, VAMP, Sectra, mdesk, Merge, mediCAD, IMPAX, and EndoMap.
- At St. Michael's Hospital in Toronto, we use the EndoMap software system (Siemens AG, Medical Solutions, Erlangen, Germany) routinely in preoperative templating for THA. Although this chapter describes the use of digital templating using the EndoMap system (Davila et al., 2006), the principles can be applied to any software and also to traditional templating.

PITFALLS

- *Radiographic magnification*

- *Patient positioning:*

  - *External rotation gives a false impression of valgus, leading to underestimation of the femoral offset.*

  - *Internal rotation gives a false impression of varus, leading to overestimation of the femoral offset*

  - *Abduction may alter the leg length (apparent lengthening).*

  - *Adduction may alter the leg length (apparent shortening).*

  - *Pelvic tilting or asymmetry may alter the leg length.*

Examination/Imaging

- Ideally, templating should be done in outpatient clinics to give enough notice to obtain the required implants and instruments. For straightforward cases, templating can be done in the operating room just before surgery.
- History and physical examination are indispensable to preoperative planning and templating.
- Patients should be asked if they are aware of leg length discrepancy. Do they notice it (symptomatic or not)? Has it been measured or corrected by a heel lift?
- Inquire about a history of previous surgery for the same or contralateral side.
- Read old hospital notes to obtain implant sizes for previous THA (contralateral).
- Measure leg lengths and account for pelvic obliquity and flexion deformity. In the case of pain or spasm, the measurement should be deferred until the patient is anesthetized.
- Information obtained from history and examination, particularly leg length measurement, should be applied during templating.
- Good-quality radiographs are essential and should include anteroposterior and lateral views extending beyond the expected tip of the femoral component and the cement restrictor. The position of the patient and the leg during radiographic examination is critical (see Pitfalls above). Templating for revision procedures should be done in the outpatient clinic and should be repeated just before surgery to take into consideration any changes that occurred during the waiting time for surgery.

Procedure

STEP 1: RADIOGRAPHIC ASSESSMENT

- Perform routine radiographic assessment looking at the quality of bone, amount of bone stock, dysplasia, osteophytes, and other abnormalities.
- Make a preliminary decision on what type of implants to be used, whether cemented, cementless, or hybrid implants.
- For uncemented femoral components, decide whether distal or proximal loading stems are to be used.

- In case of a contralateral total hip replacement, determine the type of implants used and consider templating for the same implant type and size.

STEP 2: CORRECT RADIOGRAPHIC MAGNIFICATION

- Scale radiographs to eliminate magnification.
- Consult radiographers about the percentage of magnification and be aware that the degree of magnification is related to the patient size.
- Follow the specific instructions of the software used to scale radiographs.
- In case of traditional templating, the printed acetates are usually magnified and the percentage of magnification is usually printed on the acetates.
- Conn et al. (2002) described a simple technique to determine radiographic magnification.

STEP 3: MEASURE LEG LENGTH DISCREPANCY

- In addition to clinical measurement, measure leg length discrepancy on the AP pelvic radiograph using fixed landmarks such as lesser trochanters, greater trochanters, or teardrops.
- The software of a digital templating system can automatically calculate the leg length discrepancy, even in the presence of pelvic obliquity (Fig. 1). Note the acetabular templating in the presence of old metal hardware in the AP pelvic radiograph in Figure 1.
- Be aware of the effects of leg position, such as abduction, adduction, and rotation, that may alter the appearance and level of the lesser trochanter.
- Compare between radiographic and clinical measurements and differentiate between true and apparent discrepancy.
- Repeat clinical and radiographic measurements and record the final discrepancy in millimeters.

STEP 4: TEMPLATE THE ACETABULAR COMPONENT

- Use long unilateral AP radiographs that include the upper femur to template for THA implants (Fig. 2).
- Identify landmarks such as the ilioischial line, teardrop, acetabular margins, center of rotation, and greater and lesser trochanters.
- Start acetabular templating first by selecting the desired cup from the implant library and modifying the size and position to fit the acetabulum.

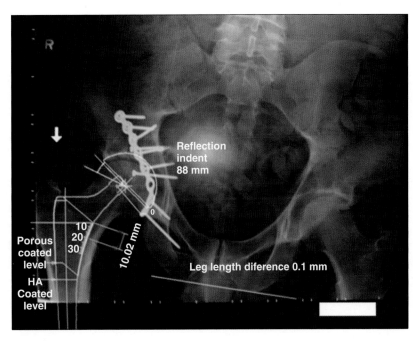

FIGURE 1

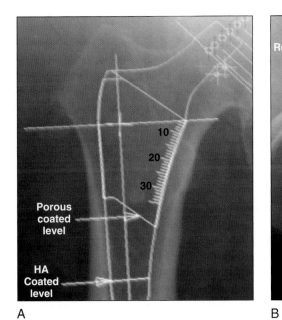

A

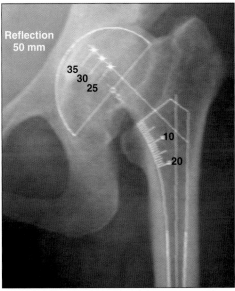

B

FIGURE 2

- Place the cup in a near anatomic position to reproduce the center of rotation.
- Align the cup according to the required angle for abduction (e.g., 45°).
- Consider minimal bone removal and sufficient bone coverage laterally. Use the ilioischial line and teardrop as landmarks and position the cup lateral to the teardrop (see Fig. 1).
- For a cemented cup, allow enough space for an adequate cement mantle (2 mm).
- In case of a dysplastic hip (see Fig. 2B), position the cup in the anatomic acetabulum and visualize the volume of the cavity in the superior lateral part of the false acetabulum. This volume should be reproduced intraoperatively, and the defect is then covered by bone graft or cement in case of cemented implants.

STEP 5: TEMPLATE THE FEMORAL COMPONENT

- Select the desired stem from the implant library.
- Modify the size and position to fit the femoral canal. In some cases each hip will require a different stem size. The cases shown in Figure 2 illustrate the variation in templating for a wide femoral canal (Fig. 2A) versus a narrow canal (Fig. 2B) that required a very small stem from a different manufacturer.
- Compare different offsets (standard or high) to find a better match for the patient's original offset.
- Adjust height to correct leg length discrepancy based on the center of rotation of the acetabulum.
- In case there is no leg length discrepancy, the center of the head should be at the same level as that of the acetabulum.

STEP 6: CORRECT LEG LENGTH DISCREPANCY AND MEASURE LENGTH OF NECK RESECTION

- In case there is no preoperative leg length discrepancy, level the center of the femoral head with the center of the acetabulum.
- In case of leg length discrepancy, adjust the height of the femoral stem to correct this discrepancy (Figs. 3 and 4). For example, if the affected leg is 20 mm short, place the center of the head 20 mm above the center of the cup. Therefore, the neck cut will be higher and the length discrepancy will be exactly corrected when the hip is reduced.
- Mark the level of the neck resection, which corresponds to the level of the stem collar (or the upper medial border of a collarless stem).

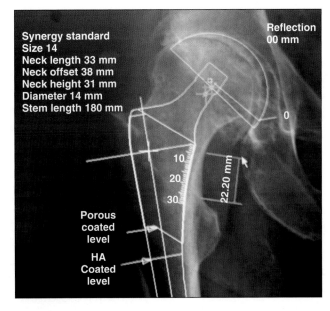

Synergy standard
Size 14
Neck length 33 mm
Neck offset 38 mm
Neck height 31 mm
Diameter 14 mm
Stem length 180 mm

Reflection
00 mm

10
20
30

22.20 mm

0

Porous
coated
level

HA
Coated
level

FIGURE 3

- For a valgus hip, the level of the neck cut will be relatively long (e.g., 22 mm in Fig. 3); a standard rather than a high offset stem is selected.
- For a varus hip, the level of neck cut will be relatively short (e.g., 7 mm in Fig. 4).
■ Measure the length of the femoral neck cut in relation to the lesser trochanter using a digital ruler. This measurement should be reproduced intraoperatively.

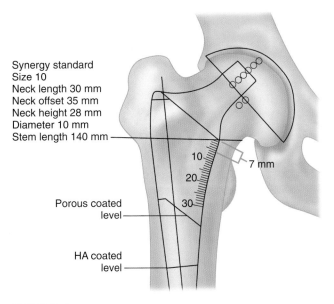

Synergy standard
Size 10
Neck length 30 mm
Neck offset 35 mm
Neck height 28 mm
Diameter 10 mm
Stem length 140 mm

10
20
30

7 mm

Porous coated
level

HA coated
level

FIGURE 4

- Measure the level of the prosthesis shoulder in relation to the level of the tip of the greater trochanter using a digital ruler. This measurement should be checked intraoperatively.
- Measure the center of the femoral head in relation to the greater trochanter. This measurement should be checked intraoperatively.

Outcome Data and Operative Application

- The computer screen displays the relevant information regarding the implants, such as component sizes, stem length, offset, neck height, neck length, and the like (see Figs. 3 and 4).
- The entire plan can be saved as an electronic file or printed and attached to the patient notes, thus providing a permanent record for clinical, research, audit, or inventory (reordering) purposes.
- The relevant information should be recorded by the surgeon and used during surgery.
- Nursing staff needs to know about types and sizes of implants and any changes from the original plan.
- During surgery, the surgeon should adequately expose the lesser trochanter and mark the level of neck resection according to the preoperative templating.
- Prepare the acetabulum and the femur for the types and sizes of the implants predetermined by templating.
- It is not unusual to deviate from the plan and select sizes above or below the predetermined sizes.
- The soft tissue tension and the stability of the joint are other variables that should be borne in mind. Stability should not be compromised at the expense of leg length equality; further adjustment of the level of the femoral stem with the selection of the appropriate femoral neck length (head) may be required to optimize the stability of the hip joint.

ADDITIONAL FUNCTIONS
- Lateral radiographs may provide useful information with respect to femoral anteversion and whether there is excessive ante- or retroversion. The images also show the shape of the femoral canal and the degree of bowing as well as the entry point and expected alignment of the stem.

■ Most of the available software has other functions that determine the rotational center and pelvic rotation, medialization/lateralization, biometric calculation of joint geometry, and coxometry (analysis of hip values). In addition, the software allows for planning of other procedures about the hip and knee, such as corrective osteotomy (Fig. 5).

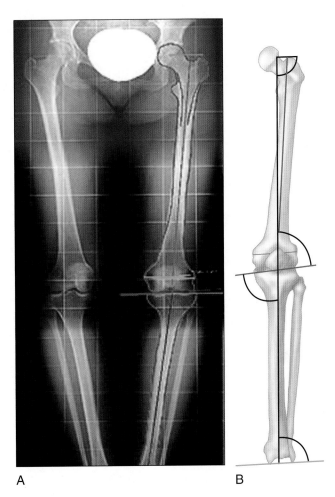

A   B

FIGURE 5

Evidence

Bono JV. Digital templating in total hip arthroplasty. J Bone Joint Surg [Am]. 2004;86(Suppl 2):118–22.

In this study, the use of digital planning for THA was recommended, as it was found fast, precise, and cost-efficient. Also, it provided a permanent record of the templating process.

Carter LW, Stovall DO, Young TR. Determination of accuracy of preoperative templating of noncemented femoral prostheses. J Arthroplasty. 1995;10:507–13.

The authors found that the accuracy of templating increased gradually with the level of training. The most experienced investigator was able to template within one size of the actual implant used in 95% of cases, compared with 88% and 82% for the less experienced investigators. Acute femoral neck fractures and proximal bone deformity were associated with the largest discrepancies in templated sizes.

Conn KS, Clarke MT, Hallett JP. A simple guide to determine the magnification of radiographs and to improve the accuracy of preoperative templating. J Bone Joint Surg [Br]. 2002;84:269–72.

The authors found radiographic magnification may vary despite using standardized radiological techniques, thus giving misleading measurements during templating. A coin was used to calculate the magnification, with significant improvement in the accuracy of templating (p = 0.05).

Davila JA, Kransdorf MJ, Duffy GP. Surgical planning of total hip arthroplasty: accuracy of computer-assisted EndoMap software in predicting component size. Skeletal Radiol. 2006;35:390–3.

The authors reported that EndoMap software predicted femoral component size well, with 72% of cases within one component size of that used, and 94% within two sizes. Acetabular component size was predicted slightly better, with 86% within one component size and 94% within two component sizes. The mean estimated acetabular component size was 53 mm (range 48–60 mm), 1 mm larger than the mean implanted size of 52 mm (range 48–62 mm). Thirty-one of 36 acetabular component sizes (86%) were accurate within one size. The mean calculated femoral component size was 4 (range 2–7), one size smaller than the actual mean component size of 5 (range 2–9). Twenty-six of 36 femoral component sizes (72%) were accurate within one size, and accurate within two sizes in all but four cases (94%).

Della Valle AG, Padgett DE, Salvati EA. Preoperative planning for primary total hip arthroplasty. J Am Acad Orthop Surg. 2005;13:455–62.

The authors reviewed the literature and recommended the use of standardized radiograph with a known magnification for templating primary THA. They stated, "Meticulous preoperative planning allows the surgeon to perform the procedure expediently and precisely, anticipate potential intraoperative complications, and achieve reproducible results."

Knight JL, Atwater RD. Preoperative planning for total hip arthroplasty: quantitating its utility and precision. J Arthroplasty. 1992;7(Suppl):403–9.

In a prospective study of 110 consecutive primary THA procedures, surgeons recorded the preoperative plan and the surgical events and found a need to introduce better methods to estimate magnification and bone morphology from preoperative radiographs.

Morrey BF: Instability after total hip arthroplasty. Orthop Clin North Am. 1992;23:237–48.

The author reported a dislocation rate as high as 25% after revision THR surgery. The most reliable surgical procedure for dislocation was reorientation of the retroverted acetabular component. The author advised to define the precise cause of the instability and plan the surgery accordingly.

Murzic WJ, Glozman Z, Lowe PL. The Accuracy of Digital (Filmless) Templating in Total Hip Replacement. Washington, DC: American Academy of Orthopedic Surgeons, 2005.

This study compared traditional against digital templating for 40 THA procedures (20 in each study arm). The study looked at accuracy, time, and cost-effectiveness. The study suggested that digital templating was more accurate, although this was not shown with statistical significance. However, it was found that digital templating was easy to use, faster, and cost-effective, and data could be transferred electronically to the operating room and a permanent record generated.

Oddy MJ, Jones MJ, Pendegrass CJ, Pilling JR, Wimhurst JA. Assessment of reproducibility and accuracy in templating hybrid total hip arthroplasty using digital radiographs. J Bone Joint Surg [Br]. 2006;88:581–5.

The authors studied the accuracy of this technique and found on-screen templating of digital radiographs with standard acetate templates to be accurate and reproducible if a radiopaque marker such as a ten-pence coin was included when the original radiograph was taken.

White SP, Shardlow DL. Effect of introduction of digital radiographic techniques on preoperative templating in orthopaedic practice. Ann R Coll Surg Engl. 2005;87:53–4.

In this study, the use of digital images resulted in a mean magnification of 97%, whereas most manufacturers' templates assume a magnification of 115–120%.

PRIMARY TOTAL HIP ARTHROPLASTY: EXPOSURES

Posterior Approach to the Hip

Oliver Keast-Butler and James P. Waddell

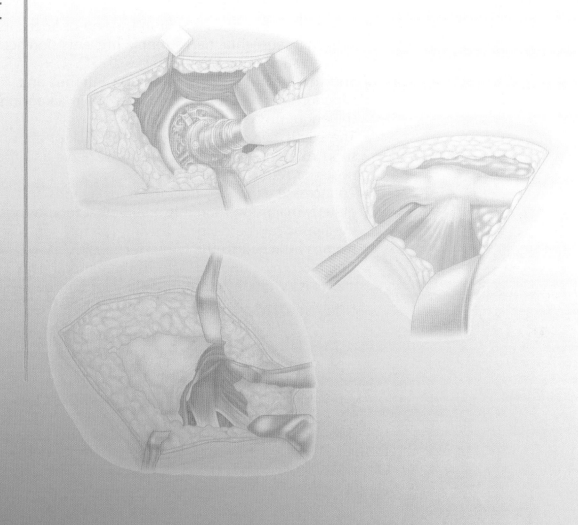

Indications

- Primary hip arthroplasty
- Revision hip arthroplasty

Examination/Imaging

- Anteroposterior/lateral radiographs of pelvis

Surgical Anatomy

- The gluteus maximus is split in the line of fibers; its proximal segmental nerve supply prevents significant dennervation (Fig. 1A).
- Short rotators (piriformis, obturator internus and superior/inferior gemelli) are taken down, exposing the entire posterior capsule (Fig. 1B).
- The sciatic nerve is protected by the bulk of the short rotators, which lie between the nerve and the posterior retractor.
- To increase exposure, the quadratus femoris and gluteus major insertion into the gluteal tuberosity on the femur can be divided, leaving residual soft tissue stumps attached to the femur for repair.
- Capsulotomy along the base of the femoral neck allows easy dislocation of the hip joint and good visualization of the femur and acetabulum (Fig. 1C).

Treatment Options

- Lateral approach
- Anterolateral approach
- Anterior approach

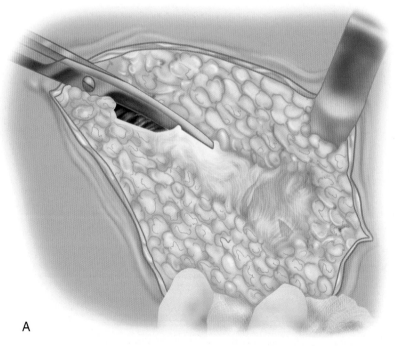

A

FIGURE 1

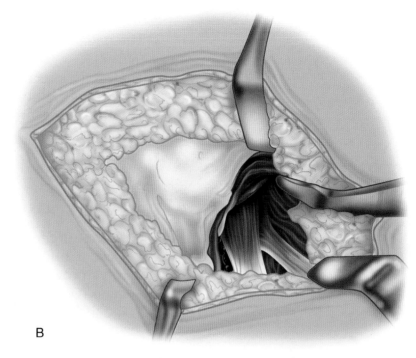

B

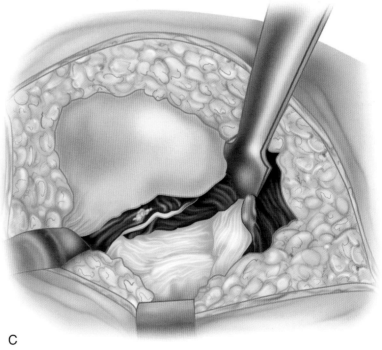

C

FIGURE 1, cont'd

Positioning

- The patient is placed in the lateral decubitus position (Fig. 2).
- The pelvis is secured with anterior/posterior bolsters resting on the pubis/sacrum.
- The trunk is secured with anterior/posterior bolsters at the sternum/scapulae.
- An axillary bump is used to decrease pressure on the inferior arm.

Portals/Exposures

- With the surgeon standing behind the patient:
  - Make a longitudinal skin incision with a posterior curve proximally toward the posterior superior iliac spine (Fig. 3).
    - Center over posterior third of greater trochanter.
    - Expose fascia lata/gluteus maximus fascia.
  - Incise the fascia and split the gluteus maximus in the line of the skin incision (Fig. 4).

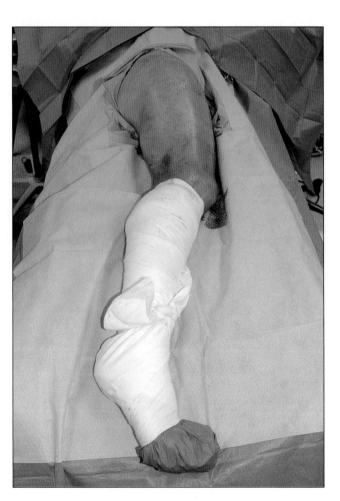

FIGURE 2

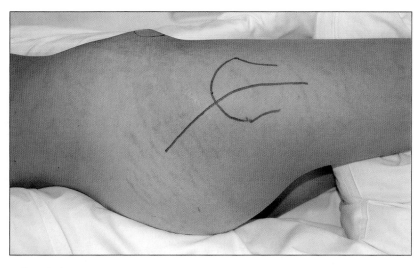

FIGURE 3

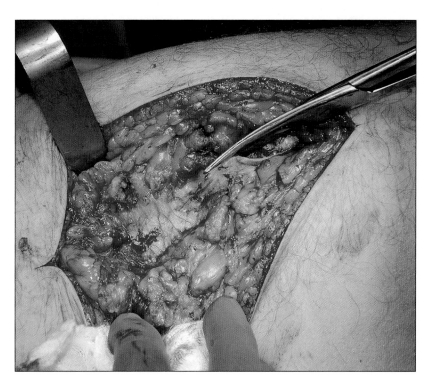

FIGURE 4

PEARLS

- *With the hip flexed to 45°, the incision is a straight line, in line with the axis of the femur.*

- *Internal rotation of the hip tightens the short rotators, allowing division close to the insertion.*

- *Dividing the piriformis as close to the femoral insertion as possible will still leave a residual stump in the piriform fossa for capsular repair.*

- *Incise the capsule as one full-thickness layer. If there is a large posterior osteophyte, try to dissect the capsule off to facilitate closure.*

- *Posterior osteophytes may prevent easy dislocation and should then be removed with a chisel to facilitate dislocation of the hip without undue rotational force on the femur.*

- *If dividing the quadratus femoris for increased exposure, be aware that medial circumflex femoral artery branches are close to its femoral insertion, so divide the muscle slowly with cautery.*

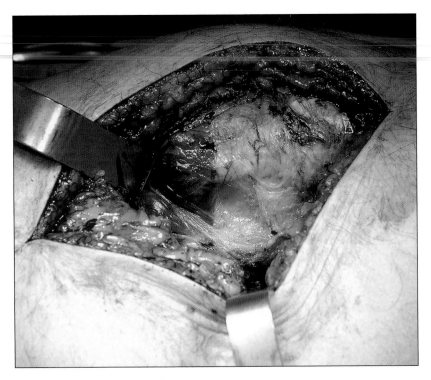

FIGURE 5

- Incise the trochanteric bursa to expose the gluteus medius and short rotators (Fig. 5).
- Internally rotate the femur to put the short rotators under tension.
- Place a retractor deep to the gluteus medius and gently retract the muscle (Fig. 6A).
- Identify the piriformis tendon (white cordlike structure) under the posterior edge of the gluteus minimus. The obturator internus and gemelli insert distal to this as a conjoined tendon (Fig. 6B).
- The sciatic nerve lies within yellow fat, usually appearing under the inferior border of the piriformis muscle. We do not expose this nerve.

PITFALLS

- *Avoid posterior fascial incision as the gluteus maximus insertion into the iliotibial band will obscure correct placement.*

- *Splint the gluteus maximus fibers gently to avoid excessive bleeding.*

- *Ensure that the retractor deep to the gluteus medius is superficial to the piriformis tendon; if you can't see the tendon, reposition this retractor (see Fig. 6A)!*

- *Maintain the length of the piriformis, otherwise it will be too short to repair.*

- *Feel and listen when impacting the Steinmann pin to ensure that it goes through both tables of the ilium, so it doesn't loosen and move during the operation.*

- *Avoid excessive posterior retraction to prevent injury to the sciatic nerve.*

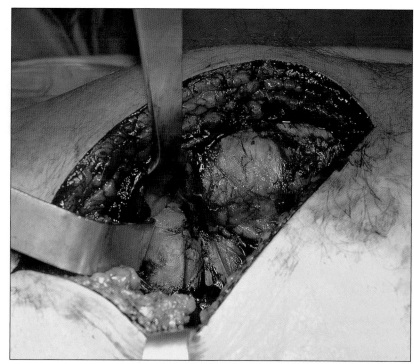

A

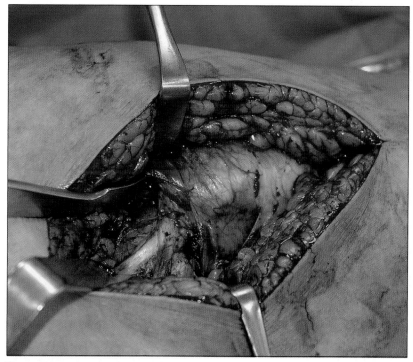

B

FIGURE 6

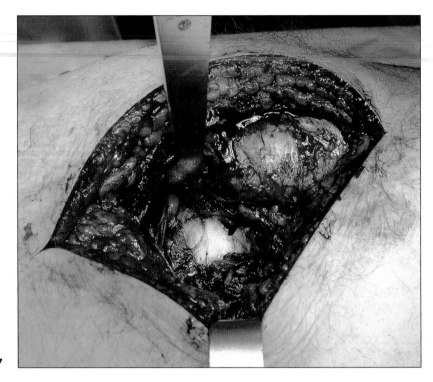

FIGURE 7

- Divide both tendons close to their femoral insertion, stopping distally at the quadratus femoris. Retract these divided tendons posteriorly, protecting the sciatic nerve with them (Fig. 7).
- Insert Hohmann retractors superior and inferior to the capsule (Fig. 8).

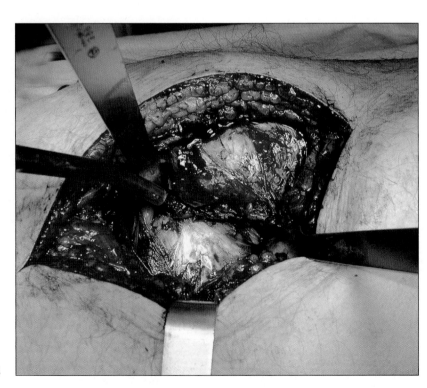

FIGURE 8

• Divide the capsule longitudinally, close to the femoral insertion, and curve acutely posterior at the superior capsule (where the piriformis was prior to its release), leaving small cuff attached to the femur at the superior margin of the capsule adjacent to the piriform fossa (Fig. 9).

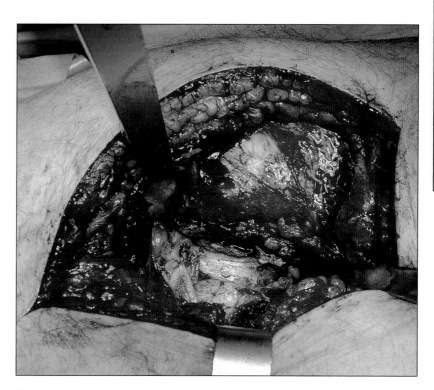

FIGURE 9

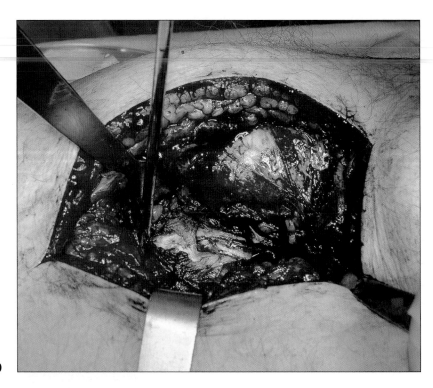

FIGURE 10

- Insert a Steinmann pin superior to the acetabulum (12 o'clock position), impacting it through both tables of the ilium, retracting the gluteus medius anteriorly (Fig. 10).
- With the hip and knee extended, mark a point 5–7 cm distal to the pin on the greater trochanter with cautery to measure leg length (Fig. 11).

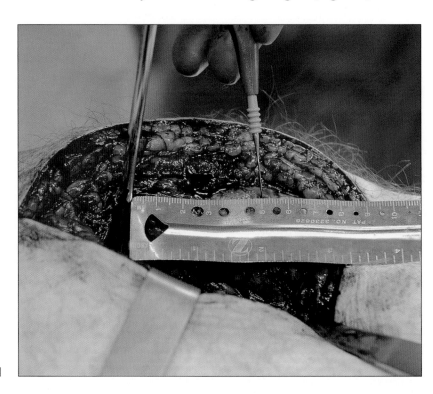

FIGURE 11

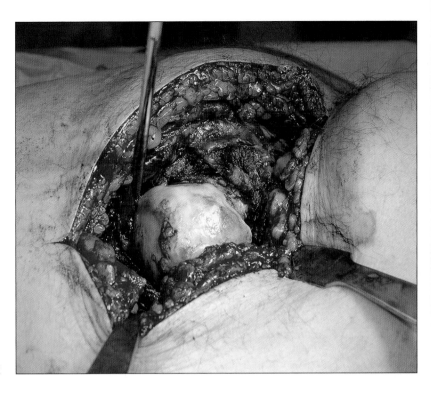

FIGURE 12

- Dislocate the hip with internal rotation, adduction, and sustained gentle pressure (Fig. 12).
- With the surgeon standing in front of the patient:
  - Cut the femoral neck perpendicular to its lateral axis at an angle/length determined from preoperative planning (Fig. 13).

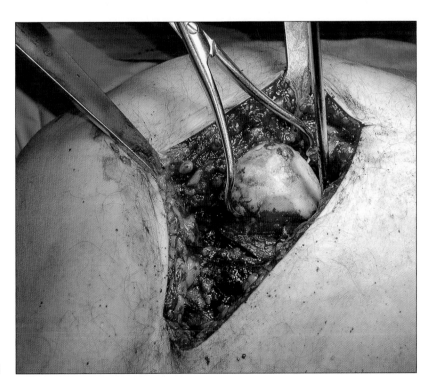

FIGURE 13

Instrumentation/ Implantation

- Aim for 45° of abduction and 15° of anteversion.
- Augment the cup with one or two 25-mm superior screws.
- Trim osteophytes after component insertion.

Controversies

- Use of screws to supplement cup fixation is controversial. It is our belief that it provides early stability, thus optimizing conditions for bone ongrowth.

Procedure

STEP 1: ACETABULAR PREPARATION/ IMPLANTATION

- The surgeon stands on the anterior side of the patient.
  - The operative leg is internally rotated, resting on the table with the patella facing the the floor.
  - Posterior retractors are placed at 3 and 5 o'clock; anterior retractors are placed at 7 and 10 o'clock.
  - An anteroinferior retractor displaces the femur anteriorly (Fig. 14A and 14B).

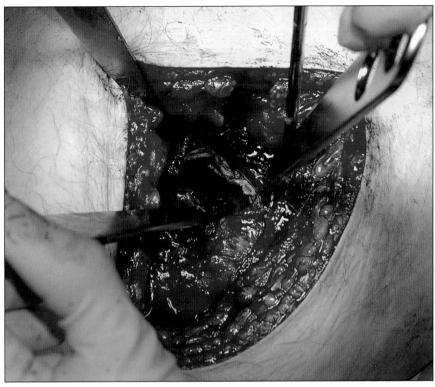

A

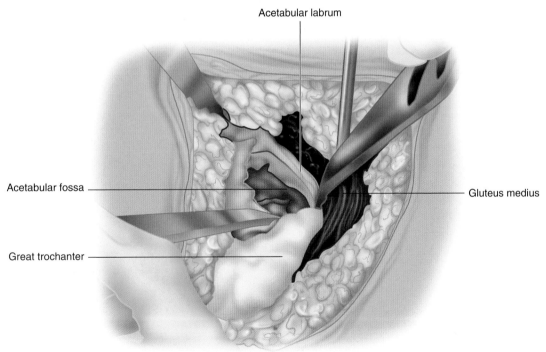

Acetabular labrum

Acetabular fossa

Great trochanter

Gluteus medius

B

FIGURE 14

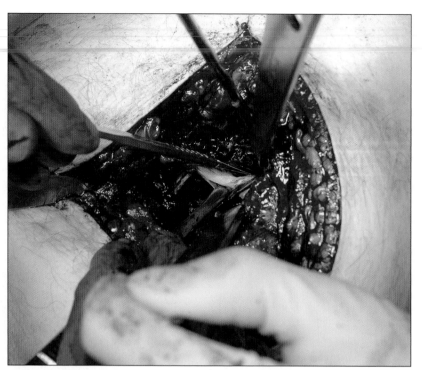

A

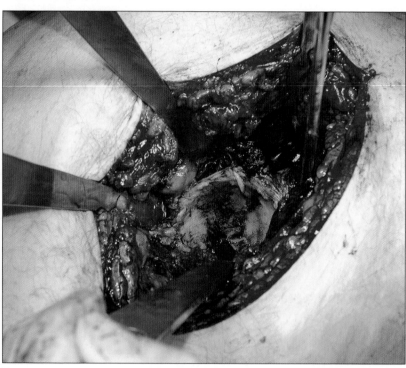

B

FIGURE 15

- Excise the labrum (Fig. 15A and 15B).
- Divide the transverse acetabular ligament only if it restricts insertion of reamers.
- Prepare for the chosen implant with reamers (Fig. 16).
- Practice conservative bone removal, preserving bone stock (Fig. 17A and 17B).

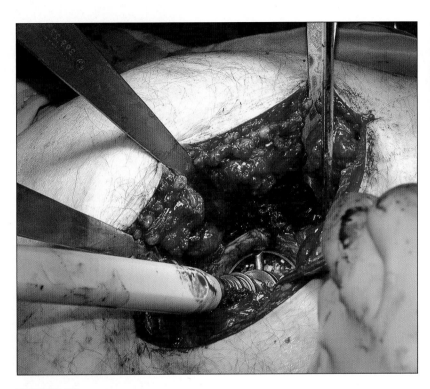

FIGURE 16

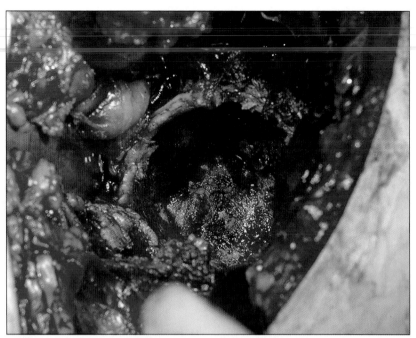

A

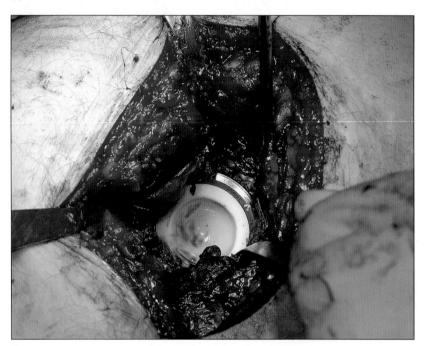

FIGURE 17 B

STEP 2: FEMORAL PREPARATION/IMPLANTATION

■ The surgeon stands on the posterior side of the patient.

■ Flex the hip 90°, with maximal internal rotation and adduction.

■ Place retractors on the inferior aspect of the femoral neck, elevating the neck (Fig. 18A).

■ Place a retractor under the greater trochanter, improving exposure (Fig. 18B).

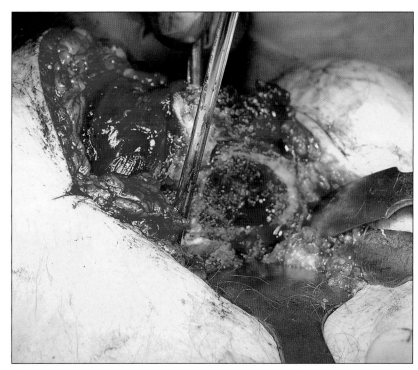

A

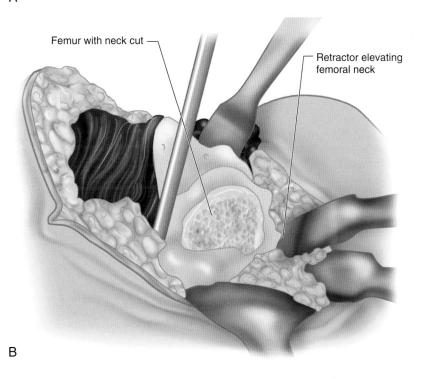

Femur with neck cut

Retractor elevating
femoral neck

B

FIGURE 18

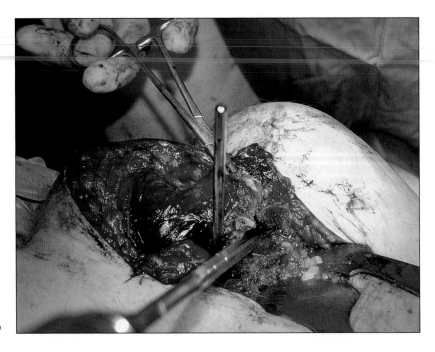

FIGURE 19

- Dissect the piriformis stump and residual capsule from the piriform fossa but do not excise them (see Kocher clamp attached to stump in Figure 18A).
- Visualize the residual neck and ensure an adequately lateral starting point (Fig. 19).
- Prepare the femur for the chosen implant.

PITFALLS

- *Avoid the tendency to place the component in varus/retroversion.*

- *Identify the piriform fossa and use a box osteotome and/or reamers laterally in the femoral neck and greater trochanter to ensure that the stem is inserted straight down the femoral shaft.*

- *Ensure that the assistant internally rotates the hip sufficiently so that horizontal insertion of the stem gives the desired degree of anteversion (Fig. 20).*

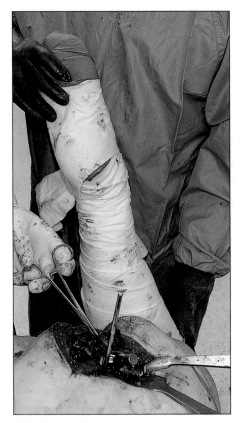

FIGURE 20

Instrumentation/Implantation

- Insert the trial stem.
- Insert the chosen neck and neutral-length head.
- Reduce the hip.

PEARLS

- *Check component orientation individually and combined (concentric ball in socket at 30° of abduction and 30° of flexion).*

- *Check for impingement (anterior osteophyte/hypertrophic capsule on anterior femur).*

- *Look at soft tissue balance (2-mm shucking with retractors released).*

- *Does increasing the femoral neck offset and/or increasing neck length improve stability?*

Instrumentation/Implantation

- Implant the definitive femoral component.
- Check that seating is the same as the trial.
- Insert the chosen femoral head and reduce the hip.
- If using a metaphyseal-fitting stem, the definitive stem should be inserted to within 1 cm of final position by finger pressure only. If it is tighter, this suggests it will be proud and it may be prudent to rebroach the femur.
- A diaphyseal-fitting stem may sit 3–4 cm proud prior to impaction, but this should not prevent full seating of the prostheses.

STEP 3: TRIAL OF STABILITY

- Check for stability in extension, adduction, and external rotation (Fig. 21).
- Check for stability in 45° of flexion/abduction (Fig. 22).

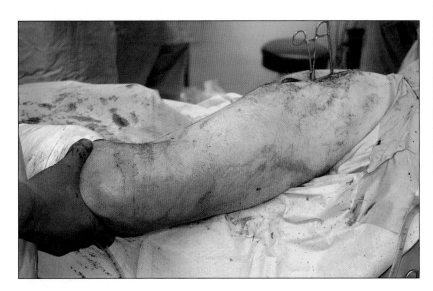

FIGURE 21

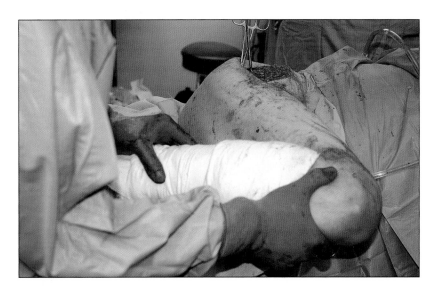

FIGURE 22

- Check for stability in maximal flexion (Fig. 23A) and internal rotation (Fig. 23B).
- Measure limb length with a Steinmann pin and ruler (Fig. 24).

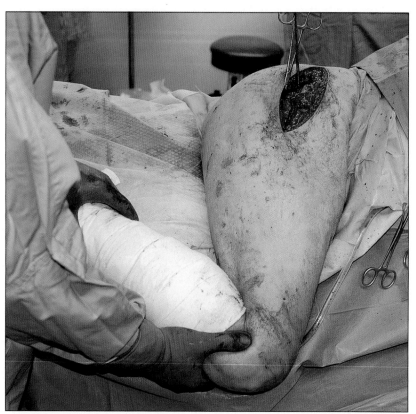

A

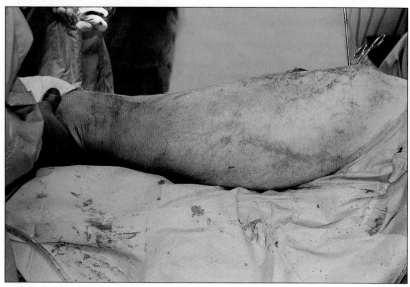

B

FIGURE 23

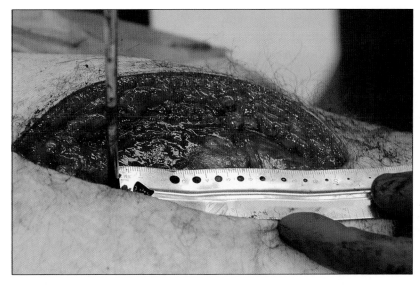

FIGURE 24

STEP 4: CLOSURE, AFTER INSERTION OF DEFINITIVE COMPONENTS

- Good closure and elimination of posterior "dead space" is a key step to a successful and stable outcome.
- Repair the capsule flap from the posterior acetabulum to the stump of the piriformis/adjacent capsule with interrupted sutures (Fig. 25A and 25B).

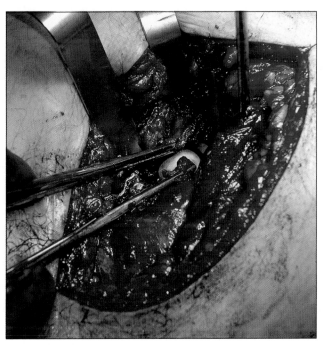

A

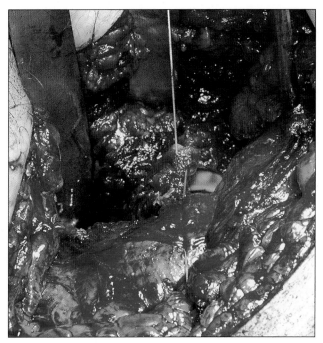

B

FIGURE 25

- Repair the piriformis and conjoined tendon to the tendinous insertion of the gluteus medius with horizontal mattress and figure-of-eight sutures (Fig. 26A–26D).
- Repair the fascia lata and then close the subcutaneous tissues and skin.

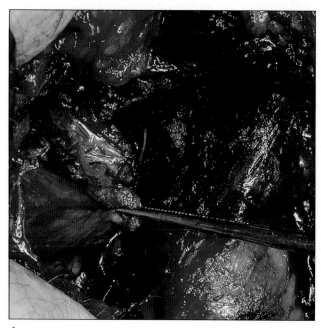

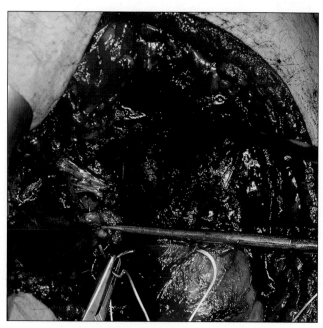

A   B

FIGURE 26

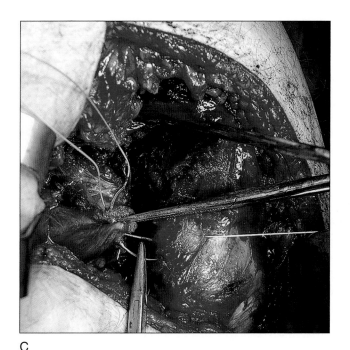

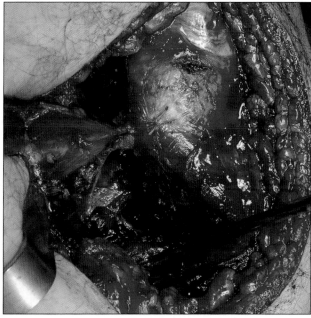

C   D

FIGURE 26, cont'd

Postoperative Care and Expected Outcomes

- Weight bearing is determined by prostheses used.
- Possible complications include thromboembolism, heterotrophic ossification.
- Antibiotic prophylaxis may be necessary.

Evidence

Gibson A. Posterior exposure of the hip joint. J Bone Joint Surg [Br]. 1950;32:183–6.

This classic paper discusses the history of the posterior approach described first by Von Langenbeck in 1874 and modified by Kocher in 1887. Gibson uses the same skin incision we describe but retracts the gluteus maximus posteriorly en masse and releases the conjoined tendon, gemelli, piriformis, and gluteus medius and minimus from the greater trochanter. He then describes excising the anterior hip capsule and dislocating the hip anteriorly (as in a lateral approach). His indications include sciatic nerve exploration, arthrodeses, and cup arthroplasty.

Jolles BM, Bogoch ER. Posterior versus lateral surgical approach for total hip arthroplasty in adults with osteoarthritis. Cochrane Database Syst Rev. 2006;(3): CD003828.

Parker MJ, Pervez H. Surgical approaches for inserting hemiarthroplasty of the hip. Cochrane Database Syst Rev. 2002;(3):CD001707.

These systematic reviews conclude that there is no evidence showing different dislocation rates or abductor function in comparing lateral and posterior approaches. The surgeon may hence choose either approach. We prefer the posterior approach as it doesn't intefere with the gluteus medius or minimus, splitting but not detaching the gluteus maximus.

Konyves A, Bannister GC. The importance of leg length discrepancy after total hip arthroplasty. J Bone Joint Surg [Br]. 2005;87:1307.

Review of 90 cases of primary total hip arthroplasty. Of these, 56 cases were lengthened by a mean of 9 mm, and those who noticed their lengthening had worse hip scores at 3 and 12 months. This highlights the importance of trying to achieve correct leg length.

Moore AT. The Moore self-locking vitallium prosthesis in fresh femoral neck fractures: a new low posterior approach (the Southern Exposure). AAOS Instr Course Lect. 1959;16:309.

This classic paper discusses Moore's results with his prostheses and also his "Southern exposure," wherein the skin incision is in the low part of the buttock, near the "south side." His indications are for arthrodeses, arthroplasty, congenital dislocation, and osteotomy. He discusses the difficulty of performing arthroplasty through an anterior approach, which led him to pursue the posterior approach. The skin incision curves posteriorly 4 inches below the posterior superior iliac spine, placing the incision directly over the sciatic nerve, which is dissected free after a low split in the gluteus maximus muscle belly. His exposure is then similar to the one we have described, with detachment of the piriformis and the gemelli/obturator internus plus a portion of quadratus femoris before capsulotomy and posterior dislocation.

Pellicci PM, Bostrum M, Poss R. Posterior approach to total hip replacement using enhanced posterior soft tissue repair. Clin Orthop Relat Res. 1998;(355):224–8.

This retrospective study demonstrated that the dislocation rates were reduced from 4% to 0% and from 6.2% to 0.8%, respectively, when two surgeons changed technique from no or minimal soft tissue repair to an anatomic repair of short rotators and capsule. The authors comment that, although the repair itself is not sufficiently strong to prevent dislocation, it eliminates dead space and encourages scar tissue to form adjacent to the arthroplasty. This paper highlights the importance of soft tissue repair.

Vinton CJ, White K, Wixted JJ, Varney D, Waddell J, Kavanagh B. The effect of body mass index and surgical approach on post-operative limp in total hip arthroplasty. Presented at the AAOS 71st Annual Meeting, San Francisco, March 2004.

Direct Lateral Approach to the Hip

J. Roderick Davey

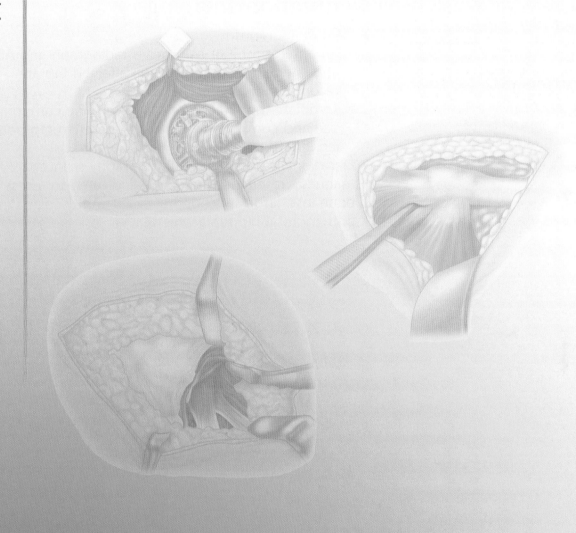

PITFALLS

- *The direct lateral approach may not provide sufficient exposure to perform complex acetabular reconstruction using bulk graft and cages.*

- *Alternative approaches should be considered if there is a degenerative tear in the gluteus medius tendon.*

Controversies

- There are reports that the direct lateral approach may be associated with postoperative limp, and care should be taken to (1) avoid damaging the superior gluteal nerve and (2) perform a strong repair of the gluteus medius.

Indications

- The direct lateral approach can be used for primary total hip replacement in patients with advanced arthritis of the hip or femoral neck fracture requiring replacement.
- This approach can also be used for revision total hip replacement surgery.

Examination/Imaging

- Plain radiographs
  - An anteroposterior (AP) pelvis radiograph and AP and lateral radiographs of the affected hip are recommended (Fig. 1A–1C).
  - Template the radiographs to determine component size and component position in order to reproduce leg length and offset.
- Occasionally a computed tomography scan or magnetic resonance imaging is indicated to assess bone loss, large subchondral cysts, and dysplasia in primary total hip replacement.

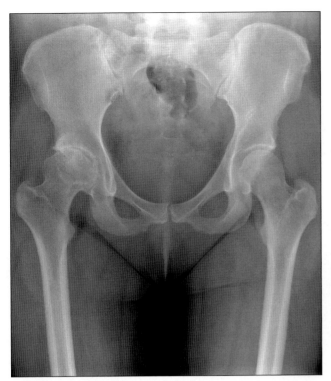

A

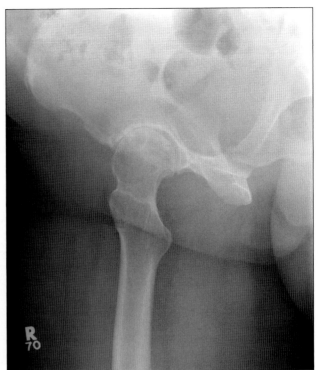

B

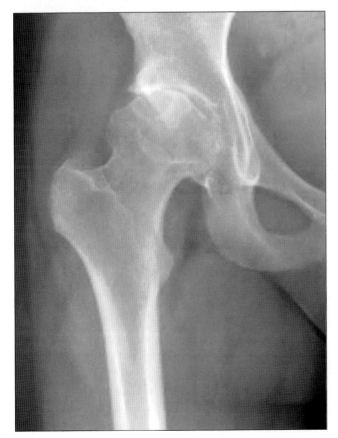

C

FIGURE 1

Treatment Options

- Alternate surgical approaches to the hip include the posterior, transtrochanteric, and anterolateral approaches.
- There are also single-incision and two-incision techniques described for minimally invasive surgery for total hip replacement.

Surgical Anatomy

- Limit the height of the split in the gluteus medius muscle in order to prevent damage to the superior gluteal nerve (Fig. 2A and 2B).
- Split the gluteus medius muscle anteriorly over the trochanter at the tendinous junction so that there is good tendon on both sides of the split, which will allow a stronger repair with suture (Fig. 3A and 3B).

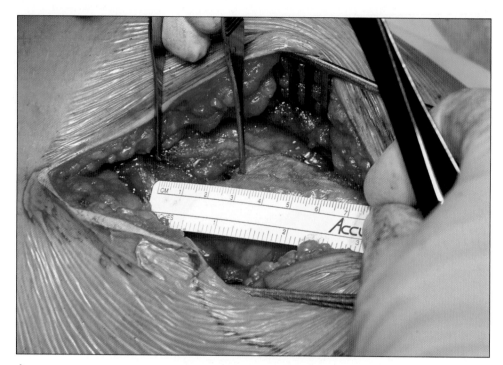

A

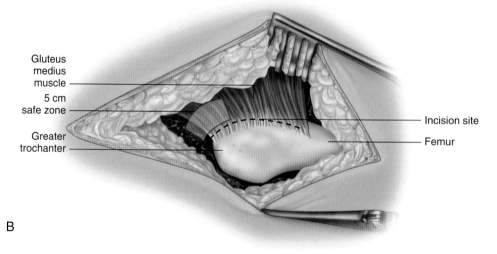

Gluteus medius muscle

5 cm safe zone

Greater trochanter

Incision site

Femur

B

FIGURE 2

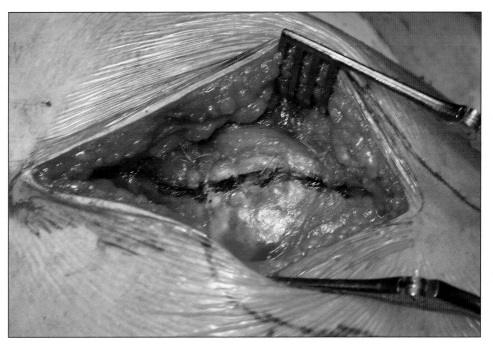

A

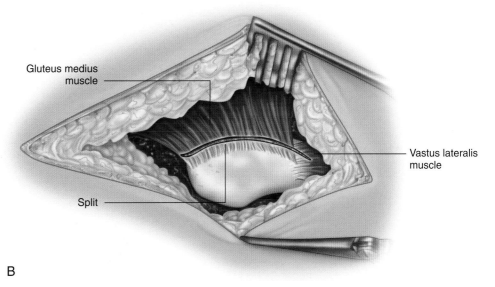

Gluteus medius
muscle

Vastus lateralis
muscle

Split

B

FIGURE 3

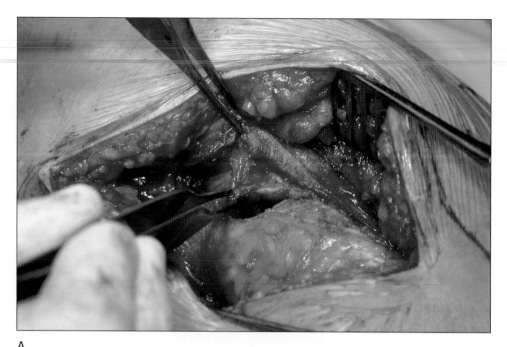

A

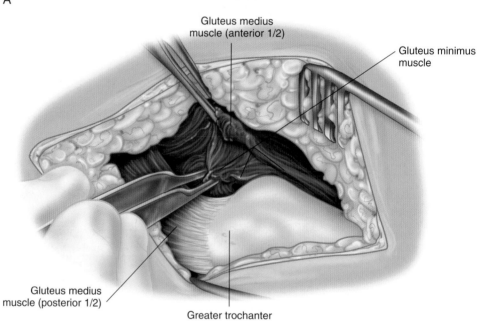

Gluteus medius
muscle (anterior 1/2)

Gluteus minimus
muscle

Gluteus medius
muscle (posterior 1/2)

Greater trochanter

FIGURE 4 B

■ Don't divide the gluteus minimus tendon. Develop
the anterior abductor flap, consisting of the gluteus
medius and vastus lateralis, from inferior to superior
and elevate the gluteus minimus off the capsule with
cautery, leaving it attached to the flap above (Fig. 4A
and 4B).

Positioning

■ Position the patient in the straight lateral decubitus
position on the operating table.

Equipment

• The patient can be secured with a positioner attached to the operating room (OR) table with both a pubic and a sacral support, a deflatable bean bag–type device, or pegboard.

Controversies

• Positioning the patient 30° or 45° back from the straight lateral position may improve acetabular visualization, but the visual cues available in the straight lateral position (OR table, floor, walls) may aid in component positioning.

Portals/Exposures

■ The skin incision is made (Fig. 5A and 5B).
  • The longitudinal incision runs slightly oblique from anterodistal to posteroproximal.
  • It is centered over the tip of the greater trochanter.
  • The length of the incision measures 10–15 cm depending on the patient.
  • Carry the skin incision down through the subcutaneous tissue onto the fascia lata.

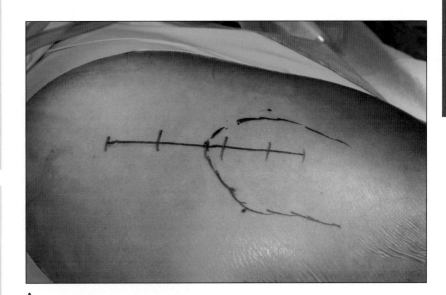

A

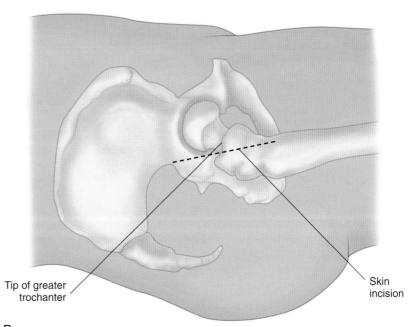

Tip of greater trochanter

Skin incision

B

FIGURE 5

■ Divide the fascia lata with a knife in the interval between the tensor fascia muscle and the gluteus maximus muscle (Fig. 6A and 6B).
  • Extend the division in the fascia distally with curved Mayo scissors, pointing the curve of the scissors anteriorly.
  • Extend the division of the fascia proximally with cutting cautery and then gently split the fibers of the underlying gluteus maximus muscle with your fingers, cauterizing bleeders as needed.
  • The trochanteric bursa can be incised longitudinally or can be left intact.

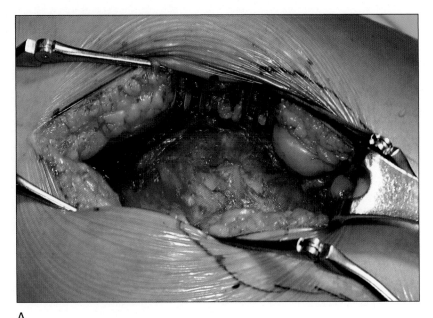

A

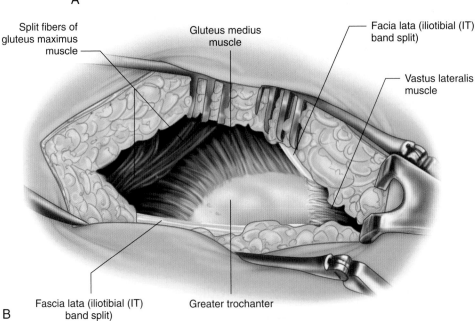

Split fibers of gluteus maximus muscle

Gluteus medius muscle

Facia lata (iliotibial (IT) band split)

Vastus lateralis muscle

Fascia lata (iliotibial (IT) band split)

Greater trochanter

FIGURE 6   B

• *Don't divide the gluteus minimus transversely, as it contributes to abduction power. Elevate it from inferior to superior off the neck and capsule, leaving it in continuity and attached to the gluteus medius and vastus lateralis.*

Procedure

STEP 1

■ The gluteus medius muscle and vastus lateralis muscle are split longitudinally but remain in functional continuity.

• Identify the anterior and posterior borders of the gluteus medius muscle and, at the midpoint (50:50 split), push the curved Mayo scissors over the tip of the trochanter, down through the muscle, and divide the tendon 1 cm distally using cutting cautery (Fig. 7A and 7B).

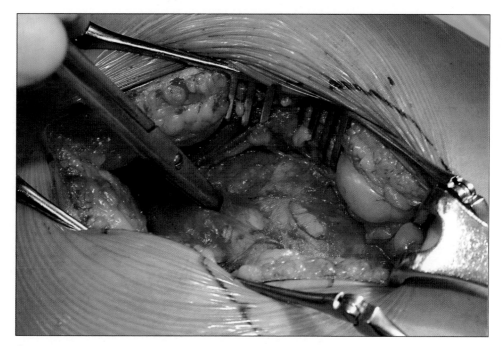

A

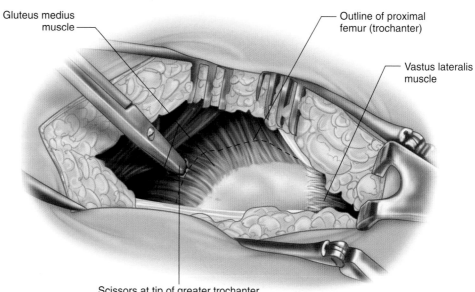

Gluteus medius muscle

Outline of proximal femur (trochanter)

Vastus lateralis muscle

Scissors at tip of greater trochanter through gluteus medius muscle

FIGURE 7 B

- Flex the hip approximately 15° and rotate externally as much as possible.
- Anterior to the trochanter, find the musculotendinous junction of the gluteus medius muscle and then incise with cutting cautery, making sure there is tendon on both sides of the split (Fig. 8A and 8B).
- Using the cutting cautery, incise this tendon proximally up to the split at the tip of the trochanter and then distally down through the anterior portion of the vastus lateralis muscle onto bone, cauterizing bleeders as needed.

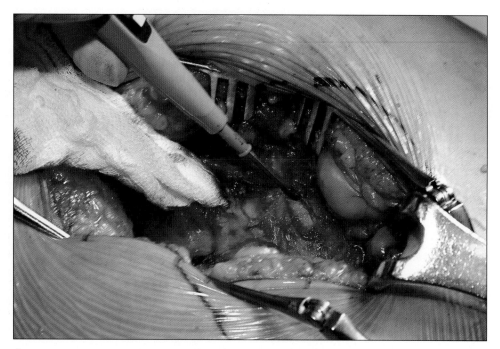

A

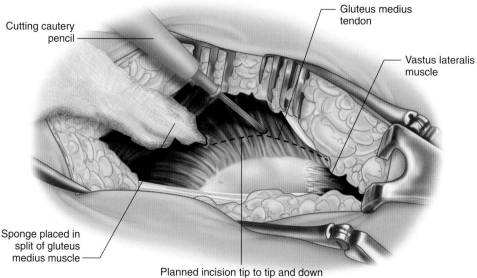

Cutting cautery pencil

Gluteus medius tendon

Vastus lateralis muscle

Sponge placed in split of gluteus medius muscle

Planned incision tip to tip and down through anterior vastus lateralis muscle

FIGURE 8   B

Instrumentation/ Implantation

• Placing a sharp curved Hohmann retractor anteriorly, a small sharp Hohmann retractor superiorly, and a large blunt Hohmann retractor inferiorly will provide exposure for excision of the hip capsule.

■ The continuous anterior flap of gluteus medius muscle and vastus lateralis muscle is elevated, along with the insertion of the gluteus minimus tendon, off the neck of the femur and hip capsule.

• Place a small sharp Hohmann retractor through the split in the vastus lateralis muscle directed medially and superiorly and, using cutting cautery, release the vastus insertion into the intertrochanteric line. Continue superiorly, releasing the gluteus minimus muscle off its insertion on the anterior hip capsule and neck of the femur (Fig. 9A and 9B) but leaving it attached to the anterior flap of gluteus medius (see Fig. 4A and 4B).

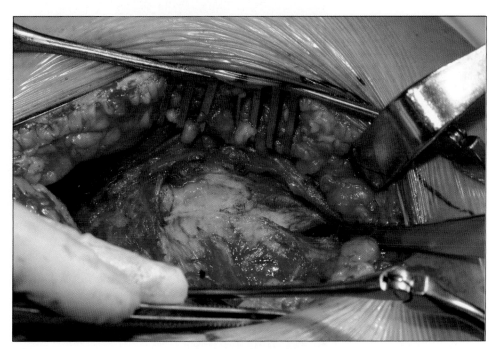

A

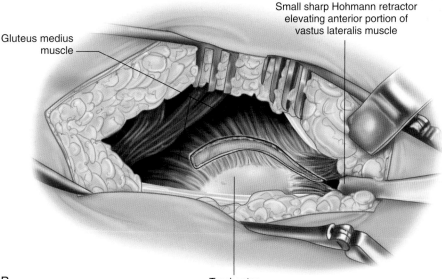

Gluteus medius muscle

Small sharp Hohmann retractor elevating anterior portion of vastus lateralis muscle

Trochanter

FIGURE 9 B

- Next place a sharp curved Hohmann retractor over the anterior brim of the pelvis in line with a line bisecting the long axis of the femoral neck, and a small sharp Hohmann retractor under the gluteus minimus muscle and over the superior lip of the acetabulum, exposing the anterior and superior hip capsule. Use a Cobb elevator and release adhesions off the inferior capsule, and place a large blunt Hohmann retractor inferiorly between the capsule and the iliopsoas tendon (Fig. 10A and 10B).

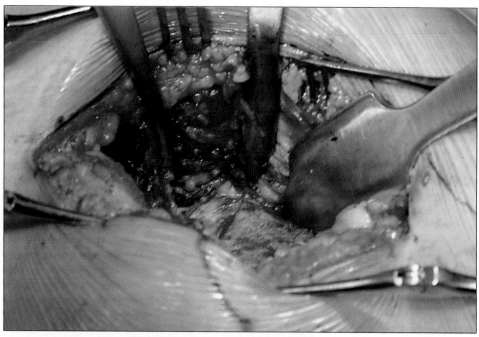

A

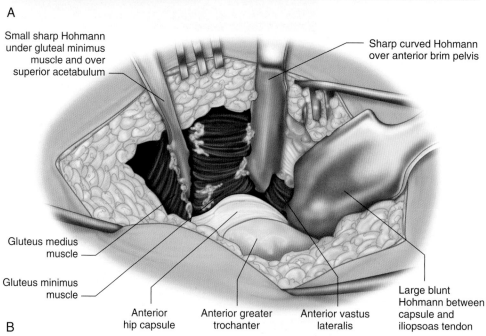

Small sharp Hohmann under gluteal minimus muscle and over superior acetabulum

Sharp curved Hohmann over anterior brim pelvis

Gluteus medius muscle

Gluteus minimus muscle

Anterior hip capsule

Anterior greater trochanter

Anterior vastus lateralis

Large blunt Hohmann between capsule and iliopsoas tendon

FIGURE 10   B

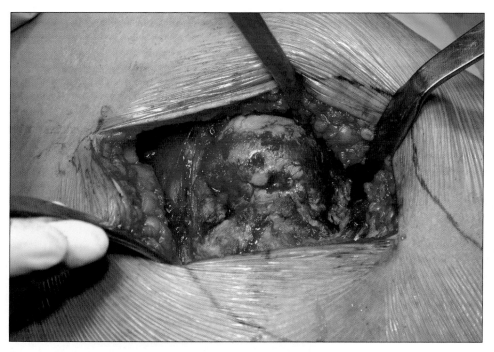

A

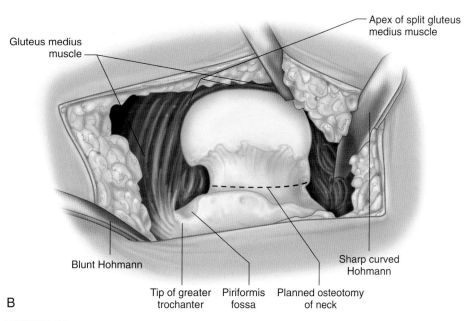

Gluteus medius muscle

Apex of split gluteus medius muscle

Blunt Hohmann

Tip of greater trochanter

Piriformis fossa

Planned osteotomy of neck

Sharp curved Hohmann

B

FIGURE 11

- Perform a capsulectomy, place a bone hook around the inferior femoral neck, and dislocate the head anteriorly. Then osteotomize the neck with a power saw (Fig. 11A and 11B).

- *The abduction angle of the acetabulum is approximately 45°. Don't place the posterior Hohmann retractor and anterior Cobra retractor vertically; placing them at a 45° angle will result in more secure retractors and better exposure.*

STEP 2

- Expose the acetabulum and ream for insertion of the acetabular component (Fig. 12A and 12B).
  - Carefully place a sharp curved Hohmann retractor over the posterior lip of the acetabulum (8 o'clock postion for the right hip) and retract the femur posteriorly.
  - Use a blunt Cobra retractor over the anterior lip of the acetabulum (4 o'clock position for the right

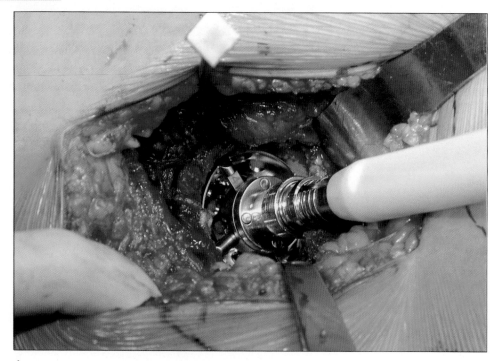

A

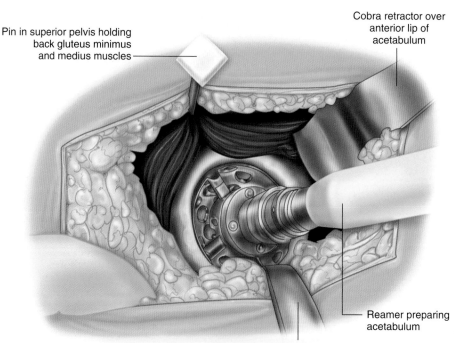

Pin in superior pelvis holding back gluteus minimus and medius muscles

Cobra retractor over anterior lip of acetabulum

Reamer preparing acetabulum

Sharp curved Hohmann over posterior lip of acetabulum

FIGURE 12 B

PITFALLS

- *Rotate the femur so that the posterior Hohmann retractor sits flat on the cut surface of the neck. This prevents the retractor from crushing soft bone in the anterior neck and improves visualization of the acetabulum.*

hip) and retract the anterior flap of gluteus medius and vastus lateralis muscle anteriorly.

- Place a sharp pin in the interval between the capsule and gluteus minimus superiorly (12 o'clock position), then use a mallet to secure the pin into the ilium.
- Excise the capsule, remove osteophytes with a small osteotome, and ream the acetabulum to the appropriate size. Then insert the acetabular component.

■ Position the femur and prepare the femur with broaches and/or reamers and insert the femoral component (Fig. 13A and 13B).

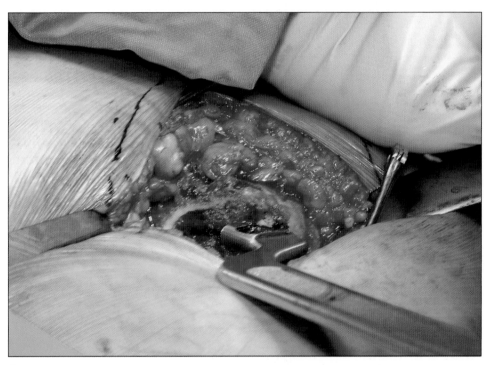

A

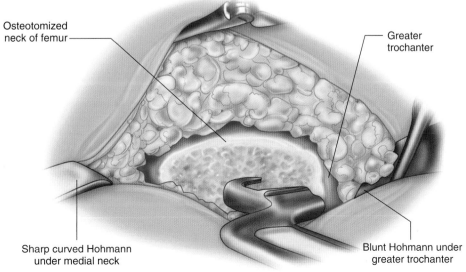

Osteotomized neck of femur

Greater trochanter

Sharp curved Hohmann under medial neck

Blunt Hohmann under greater trochanter

FIGURE 13 B

Instrumentation/ Implantation

- No special instruments are required. Placing a sharp curved Hohmann retractor posteriorly, a Cobra retractor anteriorly, and a pin in the pelvis superiorly gives excellent acetabular exposure.

PEARLS

- *You do not have to repair the gluteus minimus tendon; it is attached to the gluteus medius and vastus lateralis layer.*

PITFALLS

- *A poor repair of the gluteus medius and vastus lateralis may pull apart, resulting in severe limp and possible instability. Gently externally rotate the femur to visually check that the repair remains intact.*

PEARLS

- *If there is concern regarding the strength of the tendinous repair of the gluteus medius, then allow weight bearing as tolerated but avoid active abduction and have the patient use crutches for 6 weeks.*

Controversies

- The hip precautions normally recommended to avoid dislocation for the posterior approach are probably not required following the direct lateral approach.

- Place a blunt Hohmann retractor under the posterior greater trochanter and externally rotate and flex the femur so that the patella points to the ceiling.
- Place a sharp curved Hohmann retractor under the posteromedial neck and, using both retractors, deliver the femur up, out of the wound.
- In large patients, use of a leg bag over the side of the OR table anteriorly will allow further flexion and adduction, improving exposure without contaminating the leg.
- Prepare the femur for insertion of the femoral component.
- Do a trial reduction and visually inspect the components in extension/external rotation and flexion/internal rotation/adduction to rule out impingement or instability.
- Insert the femoral component.

STEP 3

- Close the wound in layers.
  - Repair the gluteus medius tendon and vastus lateralis muscle with interrupted sutures, making sure there is a strong tendon-to-tendon repair (Fig. 14A and 14B).

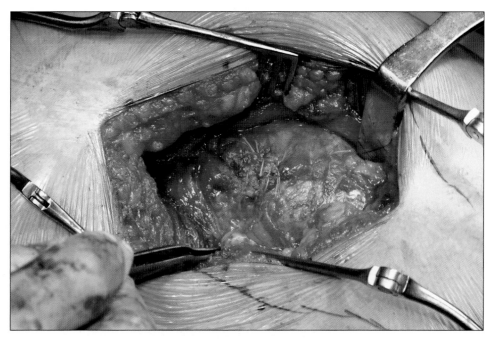

A

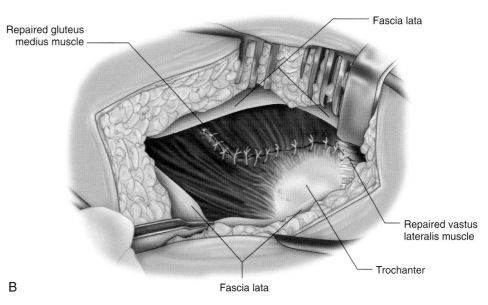

Repaired gluteus medius muscle

Fascia lata

Fascia lata

Repaired vastus lateralis muscle

Trochanter

B

FIGURE 14

- Close the fascia lata and the subcutaneous layers with interrupted sutures (Fig. 15A and 15B).
- Close the skin with staples or a subcuticular running stitch (Fig. 16A and 16B).

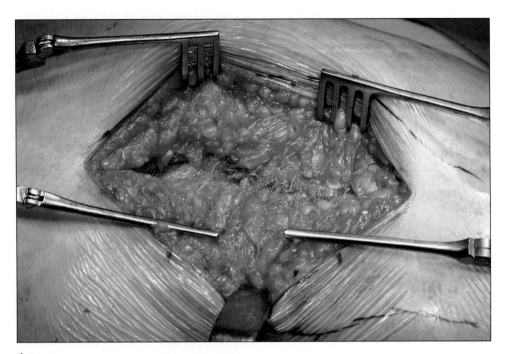

A

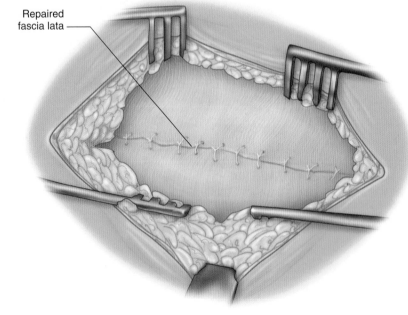

Repaired fascia lata

B

FIGURE 15

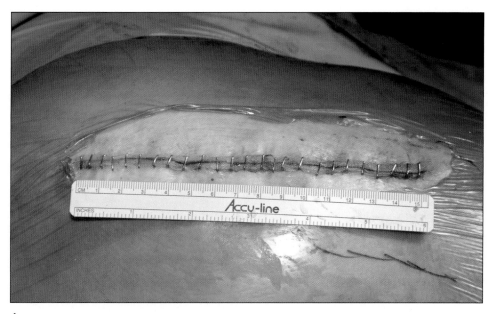

A

Closed incision
(15 cm)

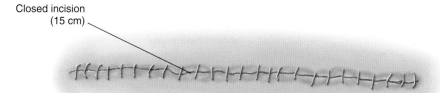

B

FIGURE 16

Postoperative Care and Expected Outcomes

- The patient is allowed weight bearing as tolerated.
- Active abduction is allowed immediately.

Evidence

Demos HA, Rorabeck CH, Bourne RB, MacDonald SJ, McCalden RW. Instability in primary total hip arthroplasty with the direct lateral approach. Clin Orthop Relat Res. 2001;(393):168–80.

This is a retrospective review of 1515 hips done via a direct lateral approach. Only six hips (0.4%) had a dislocation or episode of instability. (Level 4 evidence [case series])

Foster DE, Hunter JR. The direct lateral approach: advantages and complications. Orthopedics. 1987;10:274–80.

This is a retrospective review of 83 total hip arthroplasties done using the direct lateral approach. The dislocation rate was low (2.5%), but the incidence of heterotopic bone was high (61%). (Level 4 evidence [case series])

Hardinge K. The direct lateral approach to the hip. J Bone Joint Surg [Br]. 1982;74: 17–9.

This is a description by the author of the direct lateral approach to the hip for total hip replacement.

Harwin SF. Trochanteric heterotopic ossification after total hip arthroplasty performed using a direct lateral approach. J Arthroplasty. 2005;20:467–72.

This is a retrospective radiographic review of 1420 consecutive primary total hip arthroplasties performed using a direct lateral approach. Trochanteric heterotopic ossification occurred in 14.8% of cases and should be considered a possible cause for early postoperative pain. (Level 4 evidence [case series])

Jacobs LG, Buxton RA. The course of the superior gluteal nerve in the lateral approach to the hip. J Bone Joint Surg [Am]. 1989;71:1239–43.

The superior gluteal nerve and its branches were dissected bilaterally in ten cadavers. The so-called safe area of the gluteus medius muscle was found to be as much as 5 cm adjacent to the tip of the greater trochanter.

Kwon MS, Kuskowski M, Mulhall KJ, Macaulay W, Brown TE, Saleh KJ. Does surgical approach affect total hip arthroplasty dislocation rates? Clin Orthop Relat Res. 2006;(447):34–8.

A systematic review of 11 studies revealed comparable dislocation rates associated with the anterolateral, direct lateral, and posterior approaches with soft tissue repair (0.70%, 0.43%, and 1.01%, respectively).

Picado CH, Garcia FL, Marques W. Damage to the superior gluteal nerve after direct lateral approach to the hip. Clin Orthop Relat Res. 2007;(455):209–11.

This is a prospective study of 40 patients who had total hip arthroplasty using the Hardinge approach. There were frequent (42.5%) electromyographic signs of damage to the superior gluteal nerve using the direct lateral approach to the hip.

Ritter MA, Harty LD, Keating ME, Faris PM, Meding John B. A clinical comparison of the anterolateral and posterolateral approaches to the hip. Clin Orthop Relat Res. 2001;(385):95–9.

This study compared patients who had anterolateral and posterolateral approaches in total hip arthroplasty. The posterior approach had a statistically higher dislocation rate. (Level 4 evidence [case series])

Minimally Invasive Total Hip Arthroplasty: Techniques and Results

Jeremy S. Kudera, James L. Howard, and Robert T. Trousdale

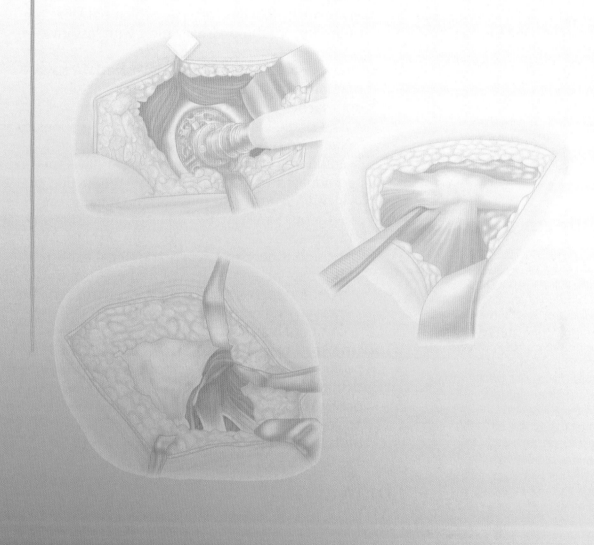

Introduction

- Total hip arthroplasty (THA) has developed into one of the most frequently performed and successful procedures in orthopedic surgery. Although there have been numerous variations in implant design and biomaterials over the years, surgical approaches to the hip have remained relatively unchanged. Recently, with the development of minimally invasive techniques within other areas of surgery, orthopedic surgeons have revealed increased interest in less invasive approaches for THA, which balances the desire for optimum visualization with less invasive surgery.
- Two categories of minimally invasive THA have materialized: several modified single-incision approaches and a two-incision approach.
  - The single-incision techniques are alterations to the standard posterior, anterolateral, and direct anterior approaches. These can be developed on a graduated basis with progressive reduction of incision length at a rate comfortable for the surgeon. Similarly, the mini single-incision approaches allow extension into a standard incision if needed to gain additional exposure.
  - The two-incision technique represents a drastically different approach for THA and utilizes separate incisions to insert the acetabular and femoral components.
- One key objective of any THA is to have well-positioned components without compromising soft tissues or neurovascular structures, allowing the patient to have a quick and functional recovery. To achieve this, it is crucial to gain sufficient access to both the acetabulum and proximal femur.

Indications

- When considering minimally invasive THA, proper patient selection is important to avoid difficulties with exposure that ultimately may compromise the safety of the procedure.
- Another important consideration is surgeon inexperience and/or lack of training. Each case needs to be looked at individually, with both the surgeon and the patient examining the risks and benefits to determine if minimally invasive techniques are worth pursuing.

PITFALLS

- *Some contraindications that can assist with patient selection generally include complicated primary THA, revision surgery, severe hip dysplasia (Crowe grade III or IV), body mass index considerably higher than 30 kg/ m^2, very muscular patients, osteoporotic bone, and very stiff joints (Vail, 2005).*

Controversies

- The definition of minimally invasive is controversial, but the "mini-incision" used for these techniques is typically a length of 10 cm or less, with some using up to 12 cm (Vail, 2005). As with any surgery, the incision length should not be standardized, as several factors can alter the exposure needed to correctly perform the THA. The length of the incision(s) depends on the skill of the surgeon, patient weight, local subcutaneous tissue, muscle mass, and the individual joint and anatomy.
- THA utilizing minimally invasive surgical technique is a topic that has created much debate and attention from surgeons and patients alike. It is important to realize that long-term outcomes are still unknown, and the short-term outcomes have failed to reveal consistent results regarding its intended benefits.

SINGLE-INCISION POSTERIOR APPROACH

Positioning

- The patient is positioned in the lateral decubitus position.

Portals/Exposures

- The incision is a short, oblique incision centered over the acetabulum, or utilizing the middle third of what would be the standard incision for the posterior approach over the posterior greater trochanter (Fig. 1). The oblique nature of the incision can aid in acetabular reaming, as the incision is in that same direction.
- The dissection proceeds to the thin investing fascia of the gluteus maximus muscle and the tensor fascia lata.
- The gluteus maximus is split in line with its fibers, while trying to avoid cutting the iliotibial band.

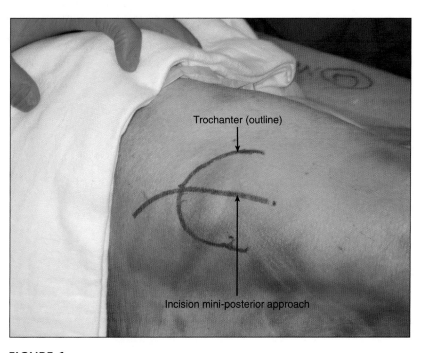

Trochanter (outline)

Incision mini-posterior approach

FIGURE 1

- A Charnley retractor can be placed deep to the gluteus maximus to assist with exposure and identification of the trochanteric bursa, the posterior border of the gluteus medius (forceps in Fig. 2), the piriformis, and the short external rotators.

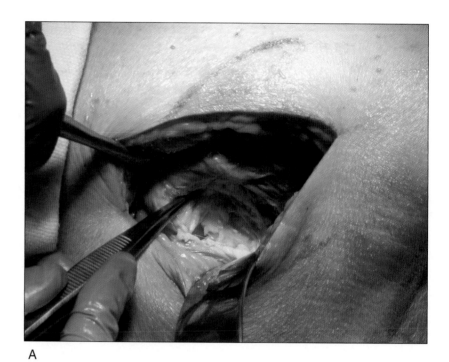

A

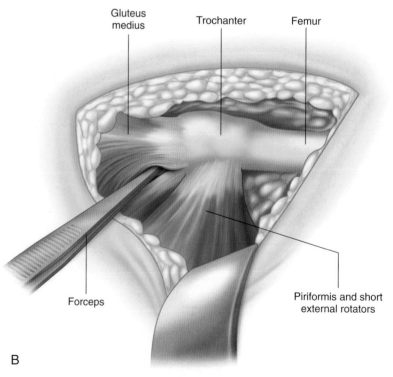

B

FIGURE 2

- At this point, it is also crucial to palpate and protect the sciatic nerve as it leaves the greater sciatic notch and continues distally over the ischial tuberosity, although it is not necessary to expose the nerve.
- With a retractor pulling the gluteus medius anteriorly, the short external rotators, consisting of the piriformis and the conjoined tendon (superior gemellus, obturator internus, inferior gemellus, and quadratus femoris), should be incised from the femur and reflected posteriorly. A capsulotomy can now be performed exposing the femoral head and allowing posterior dislocation of the hip. Alternatively, the capsule and external rotators can be incised and reflected as a single layer.

Instrumentation/ Implantation

- Angled reamers can be utilized to help avoid impingement on soft tissues.

Procedure

Step 1

- The femoral neck is cut with an oscillating saw, the femoral head removed, and attention turned to preparation of the acetabulum.
- Ideally, an acetabular retractor with a sharp tip and a light to illuminate the acetabulum should be placed on the anterior rim.
- The inferior capsule may need to be divided, and the final step to gain maximum acetabular exposure is flexion and adduction of the femur.
- Before reaming, the labrum should be excised and any visible osteophytes removed. The acetabulum is then sequentially reamed under direct vision, making certain the femur does not force the reamer into the posterior column.
- Once reaming of the acetabulum is complete, the implant is inserted.

STEP 2

- The femur is prepared under direct vision while protecting the posterior edge of the abductor muscles (*A* in Fig. 3) with a retractor. Positioning the femur in flexion in line with the skin incision and pushing the proximal femur up through the wound can aid greatly with proximal femur exposure (*B* in Fig. 3B).

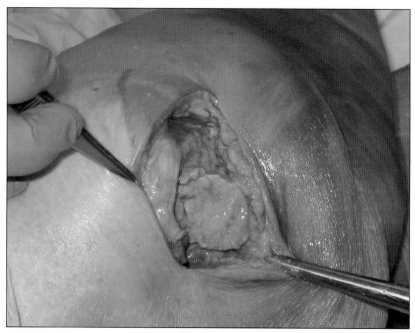

A

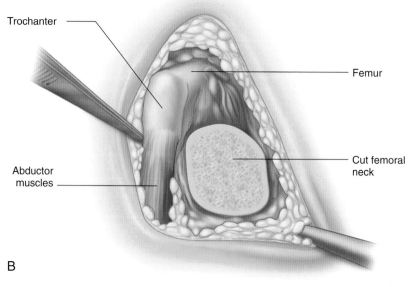

B

FIGURE 3

- With the final broach and a trial head and neck in place, a trial reduction is performed to assess limb length, stability, and signs of impingement. An intraoperative radiograph may be used to ensure proper implant position.
- The femoral components are inserted, and the wound is copiously irrigated before reattachment of the short external rotators and capsule to the femur.
- The wound is closed in layers as usual.

Postoperative Care and Expected Outcomes

- Results of mini-posterior THA are preliminary and certainly conflicting. Some series show improvement in function and decreased blood requirements (Chimento et al., 2005; Wenz et al., 2002), while others show no difference (Ogonda et al., 2005).
- Interestingly, no functional differences were found between patients who had both a mini-posterior THA and a two-incision THA on the contralateral hip (Pagnano et al., 2006).

SINGLE-INCISION ANTEROLATERAL APPROACH

Positioning

- The patient is positioned in either the lateral decubitus or supine position.

Complications

- Other potential disadvantages and complications documented in the literature include higher rates of wound and soft tissue complications as well as muscle damage and component problems (Mardones et al., 2005; Meneghini et al., 2006; Teet et al., 2006; Woolson et al. 2004).

Portals/Exposures

- The skin incision is centered on a point 2 cm distal to the tip of the greater trochanter, with the proximal half angled 30° posterior to the long axis of the femur and the distal half angled 30° anterior (Fig. 4). This incision should be centered to allow for extension in either direction for better acetabular or femoral exposure if needed.
- Initial dissection is taken down to the fascia. The subcutaneous tissue is cleared from the fascia, creating a "mobile window" that can be shifted to facilitate ideal exposure of the acetabulum and proximal femur.
- At this point, the anterior third of the gluteus medius, the entire gluteus minimus, and the anterior half of the capsule are elevated in one layer.
- The remaining hip capsule is incised superiorly and inferiorly, which allows excellent exposure while maintaining the hip capsule integrity for increased stability postoperatively. The hip is dislocated, and the femoral neck cut is made using an oscillating saw.

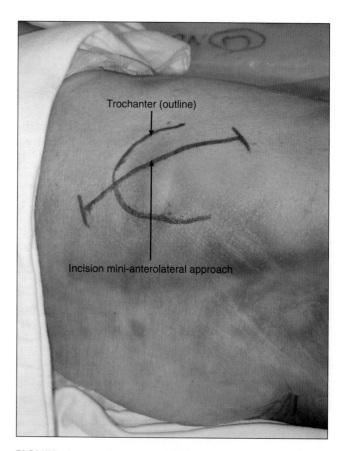

Trochanter (outline)

Incision mini-anterolateral approach

FIGURE 4

Procedure

STEP 1

- Four acetabular retractors can now be strategically placed around the anterior, superior, inferior, and posterior aspects of the acetabulum.
- The labrum should be excised to help visualize the periphery of the acetabulum, and osteophytes removed.
- Sequential reaming should be performed, ensuring proper placement of the retractors to protect the skin and soft tissue.
- The cementless implant is inserted under direct visualization.

STEP 2

- To assist with preparation of the femur, one retractor is placed posterior to the femur, and one is placed lateral to it. These retractors can again assist with protecting the skin and soft tissues during reaming and broaching.
- The femoral canal is prepared as usual, and with the final broach and a trial head and neck in place, a trial reduction is performed to assess limb length, stability, and signs of impingement.
- The final components are inserted, and the wound is closed in layers, focusing on repair of the gluteus medius tendon back to the femur.

Postoperative Care and Expected Outcomes

- The proposed benefits of the mini-anterolateral THA are similar to those of other minimally invasive techniques, and include decreased pain, blood loss, rehabilitation time, operative time, length of hospital stay, and overall complications.
- However, just as with the other minimally invasive THA techniques, the results of the mini-anterolateral THA are short term, controversial, and inconsistent (Asayama et al., 2006; Ciminiello et al., 2006; O'Brien and Rorabeck, 2005).
- The general consensus has been that mini-anterolateral THA can be achieved with satisfactory results, but the reduced wound size does not seem to benefit the patient in any way when compared with a standard incision (Asayama et al., 2006; Ciminiello et al., 2006).

PEARLS

- *This approach obviates the need for special instrumentation, and many surgeons find that acetabular component positioning is easier with this approach.*

PITFALLS

- *The orthopedic literature is lacking with regard to results of this approach when compared to the mini-posterior approach.*

SINGLE-INCISION DIRECT ANTERIOR APPROACH

Positioning

- The authors who originally developed the technique describe orienting the operating room table at right angles to the walls to provide accurate references for anatomic orientation (Kennon et al., 2003).
- The patient is positioned in the supine position, and the uninvolved lower limb should be abducted to allow for intraoperative adduction of the operative extremity.
- A sandbag, bump, or bolster should be placed under the ipsilateral buttock to tilt the pelvis forward, placing the lower limb in slight extension.

Portals/Exposures

- The incision is typically made along the medial border of the tensor fascia lata, and is parallel to a line that connects the anterior superior iliac spine (outlined proximal to the incision in Fig. 5) and the tip of the greater trochanter. The approximate location of the femoral neurovascular bundle should be kept in mind (outlined medial to the incision in Fig. 5). The remainder of the exposure should be done through a modified Smith-Peterson approach.

PEARLS

- *Traction on the limb may facilitate head removal.*

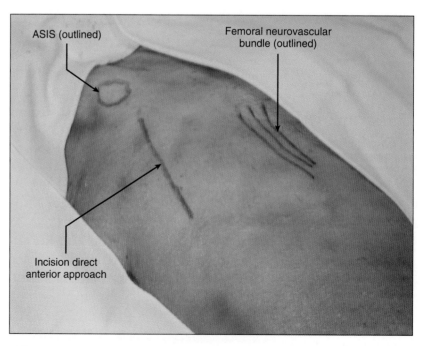

FIGURE 5

■ The initial dissection is through the internervous muscular plane between the sartorius and the tensor fascia lata (Fig. 6). The fascia is incised just lateral to that location to avoid injuring the lateral femoral cutaneous nerve.

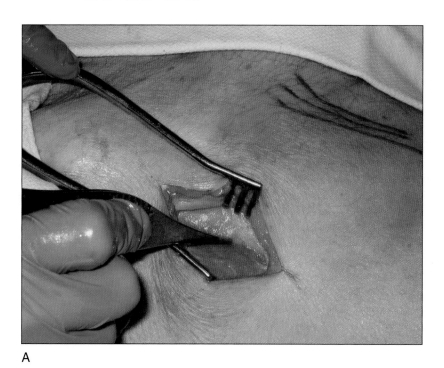

A

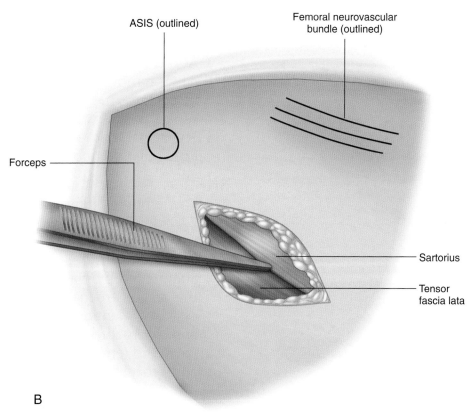

B

FIGURE 6

- Blunt dissection is used to establish the deep plane of dissection between the gluteus medius laterally and the rectus femoris medially, allowing the interval between the rectus and the hip capsule to be developed. The origin of the rectus femoris is not routinely detached.
- A narrow Cobra retractor is placed superiorly to better expose the hip capsule. A second Cobra retractor is placed over the superolateral joint capsule, and a third is placed over the inferomedial joint capsule. The latter two retractors should be perpendicular to the femoral neck.
- The anterior capsule is now excised, exposing the femoral neck, which needs to be osteotomized in situ to dislocate the hip. The neck cut is made and the head is removed using a corkscrew or threaded Steinmann pins. If it is difficult to deliver the entire head through the wound, an additional cut may need to be made at the head-neck junction.

Procedure

Step 1

- Three narrow Cobra retractors placed around the rim of the acetabulum are used to gain complete visualization for acetabular preparation. Any remaining labrum and osteophytes should be excised.
- At this point, the sandbag, bump, or bolster can be either removed or deflated from underneath the buttock so that reaming is done in the anatomic supine position.
- The acetabulum is sequentially reamed, and the acetabular component is impacted into place.

Step 2

- The femur is then exposed for preparation (*A* in Fig. 7; *B* indicates the abductor muscles). A bone hook can be placed posterior to the lesser trochanter to facilitate exposure. Elevation of the femur can be augmented by placing a rigid retractor posterior to the greater trochanter. If exposure still remains difficult, intentional release of the posterior capsule and external rotators can be performed.
- Once the femur is appropriately exposed, reaming and broaching are performed as usual.
- If the surgeon has any doubts regarding implant position, the supine positioning allows easy use of intraoperative fluoroscopy if needed. Trial reductions are performed to assess limb length, stability, and

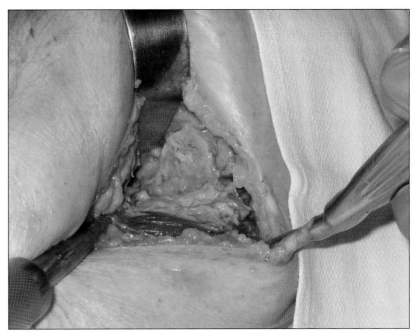

A

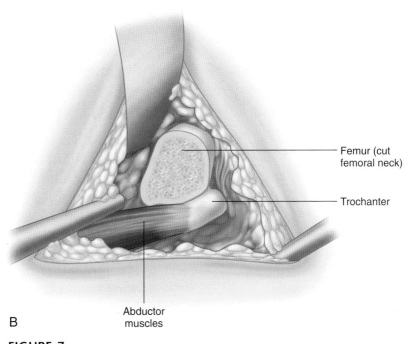

B

Femur (cut femoral neck)

Trochanter

Abductor muscles

FIGURE 7

signs of impingement. The definitive components are inserted.

■ The wound is copiously irrigated, the fascia between the sartorius and the tensor fascia lata is repaired while avoiding entrapment of the lateral femoral cutaneous nerve, and the remainder of the wound is closed in layers as usual.

Complications

• There are other potential complications that may argue against some of the original proposed advantages (Meneghini et al., 2006).

Postoperative Care and Expected Outcomes

■ Advocates of the direct anterior minimally invasive THA describe many advantages to this approach (Kennon et al., 2003). These include absence of releasing or distorting the abductor mechanism, excellent anatomic visualization of the acetabulum and femur, reduced soft tissue dissection, reduced blood loss, and reduced operative time (Rachbauer, 2005).

TWO-INCISION APPROACH

Positioning

■ The patient is placed in the supine position on a radiolucent table to allow for intraoperative fluoroscopy.
■ Just as with the direct anterior approach, a sandbag, bump, or bolster should be placed under the ipsilateral buttock to tilt the pelvis forward and place the lower limb in extension.

Portals/Exposures

ACETABULUM

■ The anterior incision and approach for exposure of the acetabulum is virtually identical to that in the direct anterior approach described above. The incision can be confirmed with fluoroscopy to be a line between the posterior acetabulum and the intertrochanteric line, in line with the femoral neck.
■ The remainder of the acetabular exposure should be done through a modified Smith-Peterson approach (see above).

FEMUR

■ The sandbag, bump, or bolster is reinserted or reinflated.
■ The location of the posterior incision is critical, and it should allow straight access to the femoral canal. There are two commonly used methods to ensure proper position of the posterior incision.
  • First, the axes of the femoral shaft in the anteroposterior and lateral planes are palpated and drawn with the femur in adduction and external rotation. The point at which these two lines intersect proximally is the location of the posterior incision.

- An alternative method utilizes a curved instrument (awl) passed through the anterior incision and through the superior capsular opening. This tents the skin posteriorly in line with the femoral shaft, where a small incision is made. After the incision is made, the subcutaneous tissues are spread using long, curved scissors, and a soft tissue passage to the hip joint is blindly developed by aiming the scissors toward the surgeon's opposite finger, which is in the anterior incision within the superior hip capsule. Spreading the tissues using this technique creates a pathway to the femoral canal posterior to the abductors.

Procedure

STEP 1

- When it comes time for preparation of the acetabulum, fluoroscopy can be used to verify alignment and appropriate medialization of the reamers.
- The cementless acetabular component is impacted into place using an offset inserter, again using fluoroscopy to ensure proper abduction and anteversion.

STEP 2

- With the two-incision technique, femoral instrumentation and implant insertion are done blindly, utilizing fluoroscopy and palpation through the anterior incision. It is important to keep the limb adducted with slight flexion to maintain the proper relationship between the soft tissue passage and the femoral canal.
- After the opening is lateralized into the canal, reaming and broaching are performed under fluoroscopic guidance. Broach stability can be assessed with visual confirmation through the anterior incision. If the broach should get caught up on the hip capsule, the capsule can be released as necessary.
- The femoral component is inserted under fluoroscopic guidance, and alignment and depth are confirmed visually through the anterior incision.

STEP 3

- The neck of the prosthesis is delivered into the anterior incision, which is achieved with an assistant applying traction and the surgeon manipulating the neck using a large bone hook with gentle flexion, abduction, and external rotation of the femur. Trial reductions can now be performed, and limb length, stability, and signs of impingement are assessed as usual.

■ Once the appropriate neck length is determined, the trial head is removed, and the real component is impacted in place. The hip is reduced, and wounds are copiously irrigated.

STEP 4

■ Anteriorly, repair of the anterior capsule should be attempted to assist with stability. The fascia between the sartorius and the tensor fascia lata is repaired, while avoiding entrapment of the lateral femoral cutaneous nerve. The remainder of the wound closed in layers as usual.

■ Posteriorly, repair of the fascia over the gluteus maximus is performed, followed by closure of the subcutaneous tissue and skin as usual.

Postoperative Care and Expected Outcomes

■ Outcomes of minimally invasive THA done through two incisions are varied, but satisfactory outcomes certainly can be realized (Berger and Duwelius, 2004). It has been proven difficult to reproduce the more rapid rehabilitation shown in previous reports.

■ The technical difficulty of this approach is reflected in longer operative times and a greater variability in operative times when compared with traditional THA (Pagnano et al., 2005). In addition, reoperation rates as high as 10% have been reported (Bal et al., 2006).

■ The potential benefit of less soft tissue dissection certainly may not be the case, as significant damage has been shown to occur to the gluteus medius and gluteus minimus muscles (Mardones et al., 2005). Figure 8 demonstrates gluteus medius muscle injury (*A*) in a cadaveric specimen that occurred with the two-incision approach (*B* indicates the greater trochanter).

■ Most authors agree that the high complication rate is at least partly due to the so-called learning-curve effect (Pagnano et al., 2005). Slight modifications to the procedure may assist in bringing about more favorable outcomes. For example, one author has eliminated intraoperative fluoroscopy, stating that it may mislead the surgeon and provide a false sense of security (Bal et al., 2006). It is emphasized that implant position is dependent on adequate

Complications

• Multiple authors have reported increased rates of complications when using this approach, including increased rates of reoperation, unpredictable implant position despite the use of intraoperative fluoroscopy, postoperative femur fracture, femoral nerve palsy, and injury to the lateral femoral cutaneous nerve causing lateral thigh numbness (Bal et al., 2006; Pagnano et al., 2005).

PEARLS

• *Elderly and obese females are at greatest risk of developing a complication with this approach.*

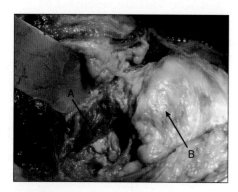

FIGURE 8

visualization, anatomic landmarks, and instrument guides. The technique undoubtedly is technically challenging, and proper training, including cadaveric training, is necessary to minimize complications and ensure success (Berger and Duwelius, 2004).

Evidence

Asayama I, Kinsey TL, Mahoney OM. Two-year experience using a limited-incision direct lateral approach in total hip arthroplasty. J Arthroplasty. 2006;21:1083–91.

Retrospective early experience documenting satisfactory results with limited incision direct lateral approach.

Bal BS, Haltom D, Aleto T, Barrett M. Early complications of primary total hip replacement performed with a two-incision minimally invasive technique: surgical technique. J Bone Joint Surg [Am]. 2006;88(Suppl 1 Pt 2):221–33.

Retrospective case series review documenting substantial early complication rate with two-incision THA.

Berger RA, Duwelius PJ. The two-incision minimally invasive total hip arthroplasty: technique and results. Orthop Clin North Am. 2004;35:163–72.

This study showed rapid rehabilitation, quick return to activities of daily living, and a low prevalence of complications following minimally invasive THA done through two incisions.

Chimento GF, Pavone V, Sharrock N, Kahn B, Cahill J, Sculco TP. Minimally invasive total hip arthroplasty: a prospective randomized study. J Arthroplasty. 2005;20: 139–44.

A prospective, randomized study showed a mini-posterior THA group to have less intraoperative and total blood loss and less of a limp at 6 weeks when compared with standard THA, although there was no functional difference at 1 and 2 years' follow-up.

Ciminiello M, Parvizi J, Sharkey PF, Eslampour A, Rothman RH. Total hip arthroplasty: is small incision better? J Arthroplasty. 2006;21:484–8.
Kennon RE, Keggi JM, Wetmore RS, Zatorski LE, Huo MH, Keggi KJ. Total hip arthroplasty through a minimally invasive anterior surgical approach. J Bone Joint Surg [Am]. 2003;85(Suppl 4):39–48.
Mardones R, Pagnano MW, Nemanich JP, Trousdale RT. The Frank Stinchfield Award: Muscle damage after total hip arthroplasty done with the two-incision and mini-posterior techniques. Clin Orthop Relat Res. 2005;(441):63–7.
Vail TP. Mini-incision THA: posterior approach. In Lieberman JR, Berry DJ (eds). Advanced Reconstruction Hip. Rosemont, IL: American Academy of Orthopaedic Surgeons, 2005:17–40.

In a cadaveric study, there was measurable damage to the abductors and gluteus minimus when a mini-posterior approach was performed, although the damage to the abductor mechanism was less when compared to the two-incision approach, in which mean abductor and gluteus minimus muscle damage exceeded 15% and 17%, respectively.

Meneghini RM, Pagnano MW, Trousdale RT, Hozack WJ. Muscle damage during MIS total hip arthroplasty: Smith-Petersen versus posterior approach. Clin Orthop Relat Res. 2006;(453):293–8.

In a cadaveric study, a mean of 8% of the gluteus minimus muscles and 31.2% of the tensor fasciae latae were damaged using the direct anterior approach, and in 50% of the cases the piriformis and/or conjoined tendon avulsed with mobilization of the femur. Muscle damage of some degree was found in all specimens. This study also showed that, in addition to the intentional detachment of the piriformis and conjoined tendon, there was also measurable damage to the abductors and gluteus minimus in each specimen in which a mini-posterior approach was performed.

O'Brien DA, Rorabeck CH. The mini-incision direct lateral approach in primary total hip arthroplasty. Clin Orthop Relat Res. 2005;(441):99–103.

This series retrospectively compared mini-anterolateral THA to standard anterolateral THA and showed significantly decreased operative time as well as length of hospital stay with the mini approach. The series showed no difference with regard to complications, need for blood transfusion, or component malposition.

Ogonda L, Wilson R, Archbold P, Lawlor M, Humphreys P, O'Brien S, Beverland D. A minimal-incision technique in total hip arthroplasty does not improve early postoperative outcomes: a prospective, randomized, controlled trial. J Bone Joint Surg [Am]. 2005;87:701–10.

A prospective, randomized, controlled trial showed no difference with respect to postoperative hematocrit, blood transfusion requirements, pain scores, early walking ability, length of hospital stay, femoral component cement mantle, functional outcome scores at 6 weeks, or component positioning.

Pagnano MW, Leone J, Lewallen DG, Hanssen AD. Two-incision THA had modest outcomes and some substantial complications. Clin Orthop Relat Res. 2005;(441):86–90.

In this series, most of the technical difficulties occurred on the femoral side, and placement of the acetabular component through the direct anterior approach was straightforward and presented few challenges. Fourteen percent of patients had a complication, with 5% requiring reoperation.

Pagnano MW, Trousdale RT, Meneghini RM, Hanssen AD. Patients preferred a mini-posterior THA to a contralateral two-incision THA. Clin Orthop Relat Res. 2006;(453):156–9.

This study reported on 26 patients who had both a mini-posterior THA and a two-incision THA on the contralateral hip. There were no differences with respect to ambulation, return to driving, stair climbing, return to work, or walking ½ mile. Sixteen of the 26 patients preferred their mini-posterior THA over their two-incision THA, and two had no preference.

Rachbauer F. [Minimally invasive total hip arthroplasty via direct anterior approach.] Orthopade. 2005;34:1103–4, 1106–8, 1110.

In a prospective study, it was shown that minimally invasive THA via the direct anterior approach allowed correct positioning of all components, little blood loss or postoperative pain, decreased hospital stays, and accelerated rehabilitation. Of the 100 patients in the series, there were six permanent lesions of the lateral femoral cutaneous nerve.

Teet JS, Skinner HB, Khoury L. The effect of the "mini" incision in total hip arthroplasty on component position. J Arthroplasty. 2006;21:503–7.

A series using the mini-posterior THA showed worrisome results regarding cemented femoral components, with a slight propensity toward varus malpositioning that could complicate long-term outcomes.

Wenz JF, Gurkan I, Jibodh SR. Mini-incision total hip arthroplasty: a comparative assessment of perioperative outcomes. Orthopedics. 2002;25:1031–43.

An early series showed that patients with mini-posterior THA had significantly earlier ambulation with less transfer assistance needed, as well as less blood transfusion requirements.

Woolson ST, Mow CS, Syquia JF, Lannin JV, Schurman DJ. Comparison of primary total hip replacements performed with a standard incision or a mini-incision. J Bone Joint Surg [Am]. 2004;86:1353–8.

This series showed no difference with respect to variables such as blood loss and surgical time, but the mini-incision group was found to have a significantly higher risk of wound complications, higher percentage of acetabular component malposition, and poor "fit and fill" of cementless femoral components.

The Cemented Acetabular Component

John P. Hodgkinson and William J. Hart

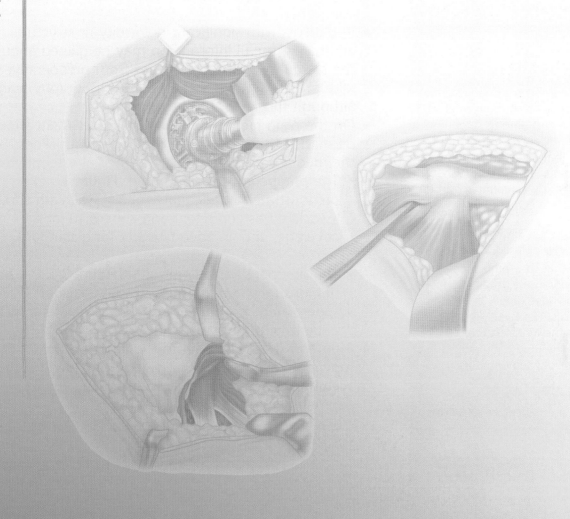

- *In order to achieve longevity of the cemented acetabular component, it is important to have adequate cover of the socket by host bone.*

- *If this is not possible, augmentation with structural autograft should be considered.*

Controversies

- There has been a cultural shift from cemented to uncemented components among surgeons.
- Advocates of the technique argue that its versatility lends itself better to the wide variety of pathology encountered in the hip than uncemented techniques.
- Surgeons favoring uncemented acetabular components would argue that they offer superior longevity in the younger patient with a wider variety of bearing materials. However, Figure 1 shows the long-term results with cemented components in a 30-year-old cemented total hip replacement performed by Professor Sir John Charnley when the patient was 46 years of age.

Treatment Options

- The main variations for the acetabular component include:
  - A cemented polyethylene socket
  - A press-fit uncemented component with various surface finishes and coatings to encourage osseointegration

Indications

- Provision of an acetabular bearing for patients undergoing total hip replacement surgery

Examination/Imaging

- For the majority of cases, a well-penetrated anteroposterior (AP) pelvis radiograph is all that is required to prepare for the cemented acetabular component.
- In patients with significant deformity or structural anomalies, useful information may be gained about the adequacy of the bone stock from preoperative false profile views or a computed tomography scan, although this is not our usual practice.
- On the plain radiograph, an initial assessment should be made of the size of the acetabulum, thickness of the medial wall, and amount of medial osteophyte.
  - The preoperative radiograph in Figure 2 demonstrates an adequate medial wall with some associated osteophyte, good superolateral coverage, and an adequate size for a standard socket.
  - The preoperative radiograph in Figure 3 demonstrates a good medial wall, a lack of superolateral coverage, and a small diameter in a patient with dysplasia.
- Attention should be paid to the amount of superolateral coverage that will be provided for the acetabular component and whether any augmentation is likely to be required.

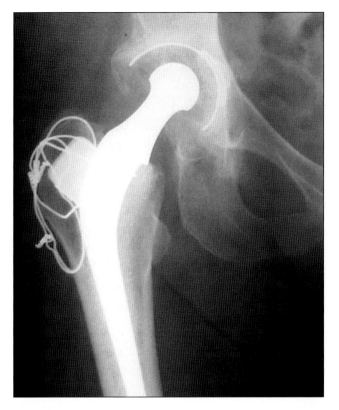

FIGURE 1

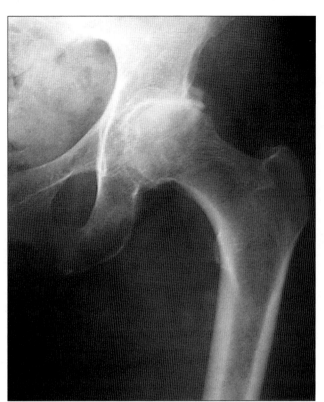

FIGURE 2

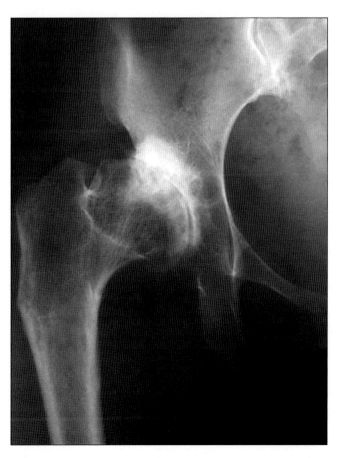

FIGURE 3

Surgical Anatomy

- The hip joint can be adequately approached through a variety of approaches; these are beyond the scope of this chapter.
- Once the head is removed and the acetabulum exposed, it is most important to define the inferior margin, the transverse acetabular ligament, and the bony margins of the acetabulum.

Positioning

- Other than those using a trochanteric osteotomy or the Smith-Peterson and Watson-Jones approaches, patients are almost universally positioned in a lateral position and held with a positioning device anterior and posterior on the pelvis.

Portals/Exposures

- For the surgical technique demonstrated here, the patient is positioned supine and a right total hip replacement is being performed via a trochanteric osteotomy approach.
- In all of the illustrations, the trochanteric osteotomy is held proximally by a pin retractor in the iliac bone. The cut end of the femur is visible adjacent to the inferior margin of the acetabulum, and the leg being operated upon is crossed over the contralateral side to improve exposure (Fig. 4).

Procedure

STEP 1

- Any labral remnants and soft tissue falling into the acetabulum should be removed at this stage.
- The inferior retractor is positioned to allow visualization of the transverse acetabular ligament and to determine the inferior margin of the acetabulum (Fig. 5). This helps to avoid inadvertently creating a high hip center by malpositioning the socket.
- If there is a significant amount of soft tissue in the floor of the acetabulum, this can be removed at this time.

PEARLS

- *Exposure of the acetabulum should be possible with the minimum use of force.*

- *Correct positioning of the retractors, whichever approach is being used, is the secret to clear visualization of the acetabulum.*

PITFALLS

- *Try to preserve the integrity of the capsule by using self-retaining retractors rather than excising the tissue. This confers additional stability to the hip in the postoperative period.*

Instrumentation

- For the technique as illustrated, a Charnley initial retractor is placed once the fascia lata is incised.
- Once the osteotomy and neck cut are made, the exposure is improved with a Charnley east-west retractor against the superior pin and the femoral neck as well as an angled self-retaining retractor in the capsule.

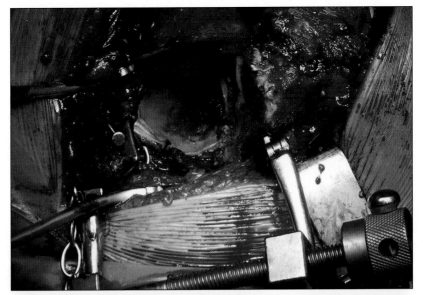

FIGURE 4

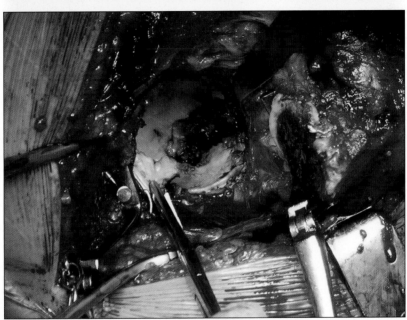

A

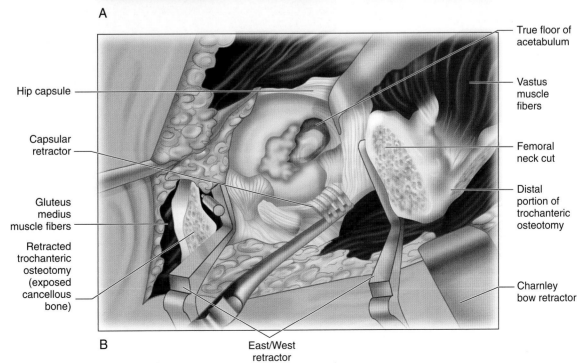

True floor of
acetabulum

Hip capsule

Vastus
muscle
fibers

Capsular
retractor

Femoral
neck cut

Gluteus
medius
muscle fibers

Distal
portion of
trochanteric
osteotomy

Retracted
trochanteric
osteotomy
(exposed
cancellous
bone)

Charnley
bow retractor

B

East/West
retractor

FIGURE 5

STEP 2

- Where there are significant marginal osteophytes on the acetabular side, a trial socket can be placed in the acetabulum to define the normal margin (Fig. 6A, *arrow*) and the osteophytes removed (Fig. 6B).
- When these osteophytes are less substantial, they can be removed once the definitive socket is cemented in place.

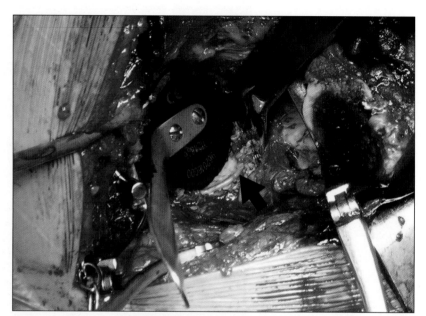

A

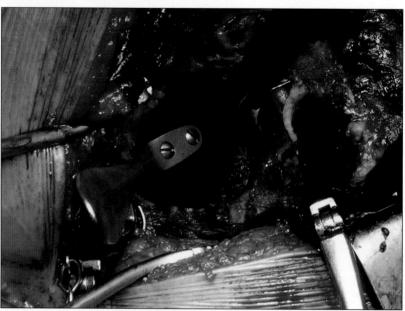

B

FIGURE 6

STEP 3

- Using the traditional starter drill (Fig. 7A), a pilot hole is made medially to allow an assessment to be made of the thickness of the medial wall (Fig. 7B). While this practice is becoming less frequent, it is our preferred technique to ensure that the medial wall is not over-reamed.

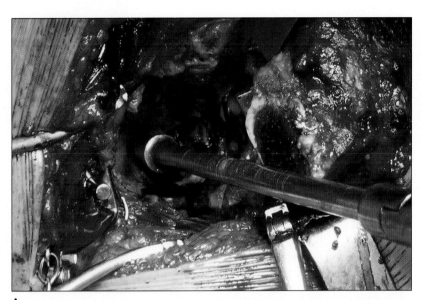

A

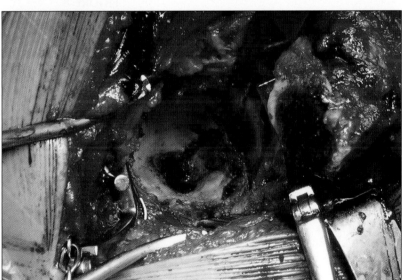

B

FIGURE 7

Instrumentation/ Implantation

- A curved 2-cm osteotome is ideal at this stage of the procedure.

Instrumentation/ Implantation

- Our preferred technique uses the ½-inch starter drill for the medial pilot hole. The defect is covered with a central mesh as originally described by Charnley.
- Others advocate the use of a 2-mm drill and a depth gauge to avoid cement penetration medially.

PEARLS

- *With good-quality, sharp hemispherical reamers, it is possible to achieve even expansion of the cavity quite easily by hand. Many surgeons tend to favor power reaming; however, blunted reamers tend to skip on the bone surface and perform less effectively. There is a surprising amount of proprioceptive feedback possible with hand reaming, and we recommend this technique.*

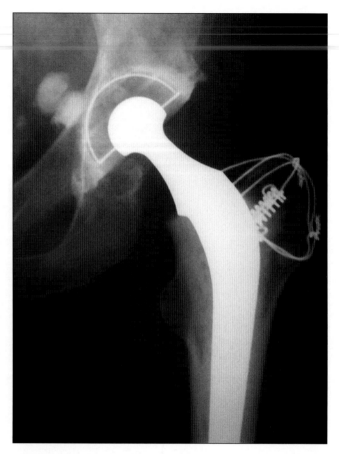

FIGURE 8

- The presence of a medial "collar stud" of cement (Fig. 8) has been thought to be advantageous in resisting migration superolaterally.

STEP 4

- A small hemispherical reamer is then used, and the direction of reaming is deliberately angled medially (Fig. 9) and forcibly kept inferior at the level of the transverse acetabular ligament.
- Care is taken at this time to ensure that the true floor is identified (Fig. 10) and that any medial osteophyte is removed.

STEP 5

- After this, reaming is simply a process of expanding this cavity (Fig. 11), taking care not to overmedialize and ream through the medial wall.
- Attention should be paid to ensure that expansion is taking place evenly in the AP plane. This will avoid inadvertently reaming out one of the walls.

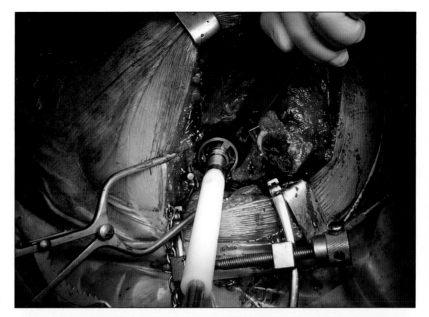

FIGURE 9

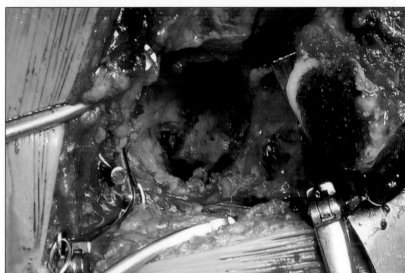

FIGURE 10

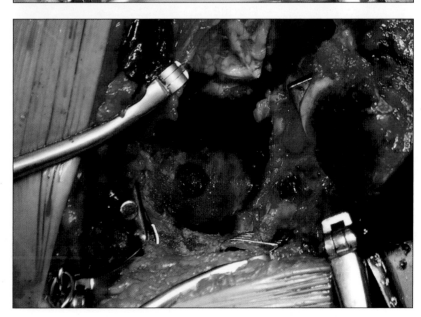

FIGURE 11

Instrumentation/Implantation

- A mixture of curette spoons, a ring curette, and a set of gouges are ideal for hand finishing the acetabulum and to clear the last tissue remnants.

STEP 6

- Much has been written about the shape of the acetabulum, and clearly it is not hemispherical. Early acknowledgment of this fact is vital to avoid over-reaming and excessive bone loss in the anterior and posterior walls.
- A point will be reached at which the reamer fits the acetabulum well in the AP plane and all articular cartilage is removed from these surfaces.
- Attention should then be turned to the superolateral margin of the acetabulum (Fig. 12) to ensure that there is no residual cartilaginous or soft tissue material present. Failure to do so tends to give rise to the telltale lucent line in Charnley and Delee zone 1 on the postoperative radiograph (Fig. 13).
- Using a combination of gauges and curettes, this area can be well cleared.

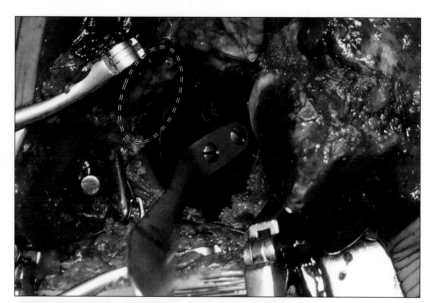

FIGURE 12

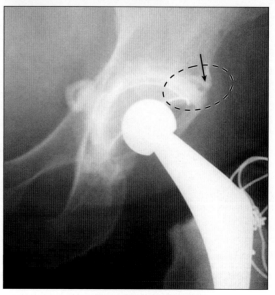

FIGURE 13

STEP 7

- Multiple keyholes are prepared in the acetabular bone using a power drill (Fig. 14A and 14B).
- Historically the large ½-inch starter drill was used for pubic, ischial, and iliac keyholes. We now favor multiple ¼-inch holes throughout the acetabulum with care taken medially.

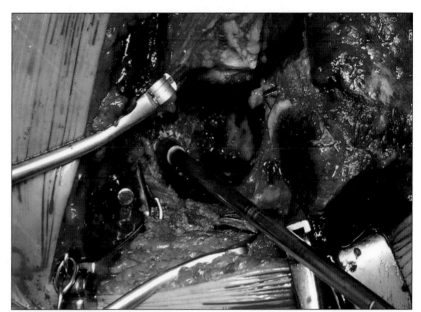

A

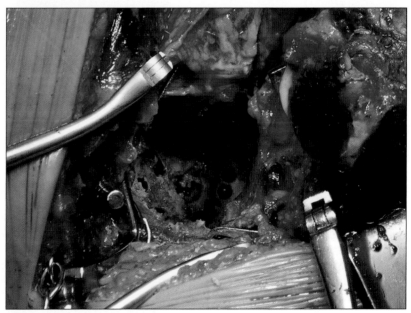

B

FIGURE 14

PEARLS

- *Rehearsal of the implanting maneuver and awareness of the final resting position of the implant are the most important factors at this stage.*

- *An excessive residual flange may hamper correct seating of the prosthesis.*

PITFALLS

- *The most common error is inadequate medialization of the socket on insertion; it is important to approach implantation as two moves:*

  - *First, adequate medially directed pressure with the socket held closed on the holder*

  - *Second, gradual introduction of the correct inclination and anteversion once the socket is medialized*

STEP 8

- The socket is sized so that its outer diameter is within 10 mm of the largest reamer used.
- The flange is cut to ensure that, when a trial is performed, the flange sits evenly on the acetabular margin (Fig. 15).
- The final position of the socket holder is tested to ensure that the definitive component is correctly seated (Fig. 16).
- While the cement is being mixed, the cavity is washed and prepared with hydrogen peroxide immediately prior to cementation. This results in a dry field that allows good cement penetration.

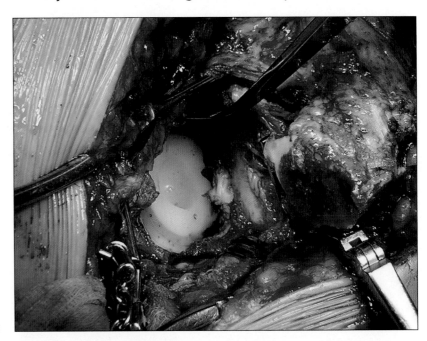

FIGURE 15

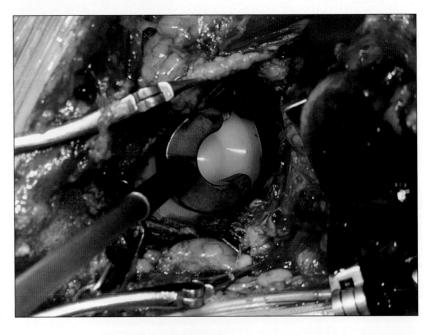

FIGURE 16

STEP 9

- First, the medial cement restrictor is inserted with a small amount of cement on its deep surface to hold it in place.
- While proprietary cement pressurizers are available for the next part of the procedure, in vitro studies using the socket illustrated have demonstrated that the pressure achieved with this well-fitting flange is comparable to that of an acetabular pressurizer. Our preference is to insert the cement as a ball into the acetabulum, gently thumb it toward the superior part of the acetabulum, and then clear the cement inferiorly to allow accurate placement of the socket.
- The socket is then introduced as rehearsed with the socket holder and a socket pusher.
- Once the final position is achieved, the socket holder is removed, leaving the pusher in place. Further pressure is then applied to the flange at its margin until the cement has cured (Fig. 17). Note that, once the cement has cured, a thin film of blood is apparent beneath the flange.
- The inferior retractor is removed at this time to avoid inadvertent fixation of this device with cement. Care should be taken to avoid excessive changes in position as the cement is curing.

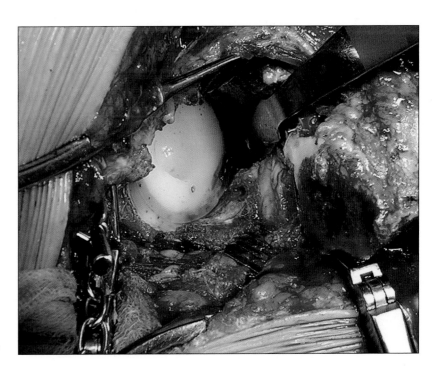

FIGURE 17

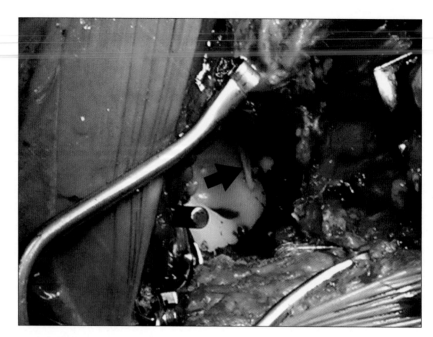

FIGURE 18

- Finally, once the cement has cured, the margin of the acetabulum should be inspected to look for residual fragments of cement that may get into the articulation and lead to excess wear (Fig. 18). Again, attention should be paid to the bony margin of the acetabulum and excessive osteophytes should be removed.
- The aim is for a neutral or slightly anteverted socket with an inclination/angle opening laterally of approximately 40°.

Postoperative Care and Expected Outcomes

- In cases where a cemented acetabular component has been chosen, patients are usually encouraged to start full weight bearing on the operated side in the early post-operative period.
- Where a more complex acetabular reconstruction has been necessary with either structural or morcellised allograft, a period of partial weight bearing is encouraged postoperatively. In cases where a trochanteric osteotomy has been employed, protected weight bearing is encouraged for 12 weeks.
- With care and attention to detail, it is extremely unusual to encounter problems relating to a

cemented acetabular component in the early post-operative period. The chance of incorrect positioning of the component should be minimized by correct rehearsal of the insertion maneuver. Attention to removing cement debris from the margin of the component should ensure that no retained cement fragments will get into the bearing.

■ Radiological follow-up is recommended at one year and every fifth postoperative year routinely to look for signs of wear and progressive lucencies affecting the acetabular component.

Evidence

Levy BA, Berry DJ, Pagnano MW. Long-term survivorship of cemented all polyethylene acetabular components in patients >75 years of age. J Arthroplasy. 2000;15:461–7.

Average follow-up for this series was 8.9 years. Despite the fact that over time many of the original cohort had died, no patient had required revision of an acetabular component for aseptic loosening. This paper demonstrates that survivorship free from revision can be expected with this choice of implant.

Williams HD, Browne G, Gie GA, Ling RS, Timperley AJ, Wendover NA. The Exeter universal cemented femoral component at 8–12 years. A study of the first 325 hips. J Bone Joint Surg Br. 2002;84:324–34.

Three hundred twenty-five hip replacements performed by surgeons of varying levels of experience followed up at a minimum of 8 years. With revision of the acetabular component for aseptic loosening, the survivorship was 96.86% (95% CI 93.1 to 98.9).

The fall from grace of the cemented acetabular component seems to have stemmed from perceived poorer outcomes relating to younger patients. Diagnoses such as ddh and avn tend to produce patients with single joint pathology who will test their arthroplasties more rigorously. The wish to take advantage of larger bearings is certainly not advantageous to any form of polyethylene acetabulum regardless of the means of fixation. The advent of potentially more wear resistant bearing combinations in these cases has greatly increased the options available to the joint replacement surgeon. We would still advocate the use of this acetabular bearing for a large proportion of our routine workload, but we would not routinely consider bearing sizes above 28 mm in any but the most frail patients.

The Cemented Femoral Stem

John H. Franklin and Henrik Malchau

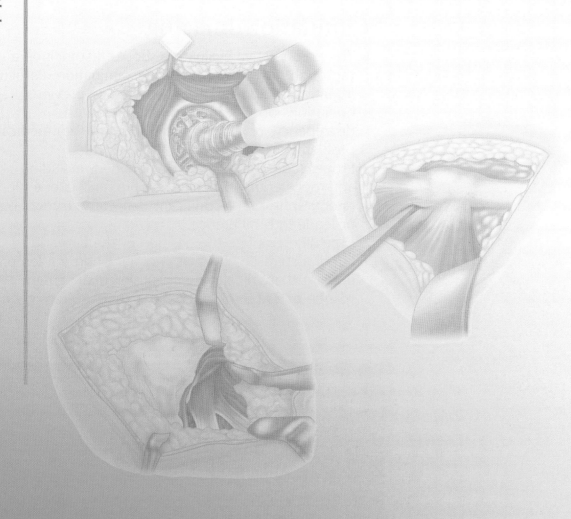

Indications

- Relative indications for a cemented femoral stem include:
  - Smaller, less active patients
  - Dorr type C femoral canals
  - Osteopenic bone
  - Prior sepsis in which the use of antibiotic-impregnated cement is desired

Examination/Imaging

- The preoperative evaluation should first include a thorough history and physical examination. Particular attention should be given to note any previous operations on the affected hip, leg length discrepancy, or history of cardiopulmonary medical problems.
- Proper radiographs must be obtained, including anteroposterior (AP) pelvis, AP hip, and lateral hip radiographs. Note significant deformity, osteopenia, or leg length difference.
- Carefully template the position of the cup and femoral stem on all views (Fig. 1). Choose a femoral implant that will allow a circumferential cement mantle of 2–3 mm.

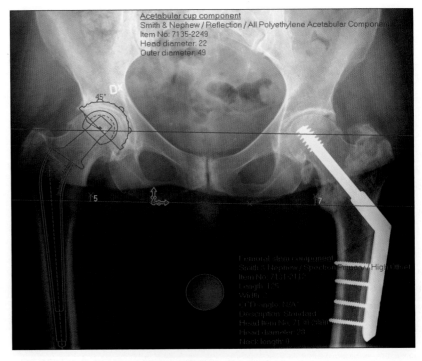

FIGURE 1

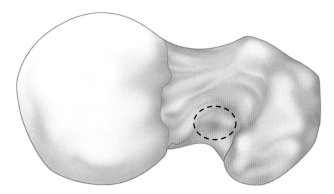

FIGURE 2

Surgical Anatomy

- A key landmark for the femoral neck osteotomy is the lesser trochanter. This cut is typically made 1.5–2 cm proximal to the lesser trochanter.
- The piriformis fossa (Fig. 2) is the anatomic starting point for entry of the femoral stem into the canal, and its identification is critical for producing a well-aligned implant with a good cement mantle.

Positioning

- Hypotensive anesthesia improves visualization by reducing blood loss during the operation and facilitates excellent cement-bone interdigitation by minimizing back-bleeding from the cancellous bony surface of the proximal femur.
- Regardless of approach, the patient should be positioned directly lateral on the operating table. If the table position changes during the operation, the surgeon must be cognizant of the position of the patient's pelvis throughout the operation.

Portals/Exposures

- The procedure may be done through the posterolateral, anterolateral, direct lateral, or transtrochanteric approach.

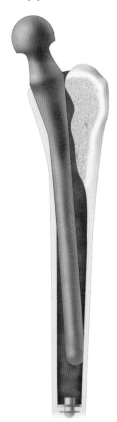

FIGURE 3

Procedure

STEP 1: FEMORAL HEAD RESECTION

- Preoperative planning and templating should guide selection of the level for the femoral neck osteotomy.
- The level of the osteotomy is marked using the femoral neck osteotomy guide (Fig. 4).

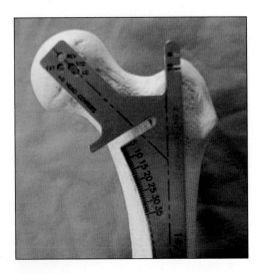

FIGURE 4

Step 2: Opening the Medullary Canal

- Open the medullary canal through the cortical bone overlying the piriformis fossa using a trocar awl or rongeur.
- Working posterolaterally will allow proper placement of the femoral stem by allowing the most direct path to the femoral diaphysis.
- A T-handle canal finder is inserted into the proximal femur to a depth that approximates the length of the femoral stem. Care is taken to insert the instrument through the same posterolateral starting point, and it should pass easily into the femur.

Step 3: Preparation of the Proximal Femur

- Bone overlying the lateral femoral neck and any medial bone of the greater trochanter impeding direct passage to the femoral canal is removed with a box osteotome (Fig. 5A and 5B). Alternatively, a lateralizing reamer may be used to accomplish this.

PITFALLS

- *Failure to remove this lateral bone will result in medial placement of the femoral stem and varus alignment.*

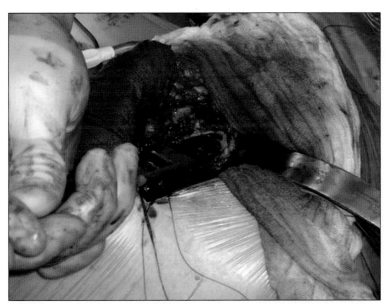

A

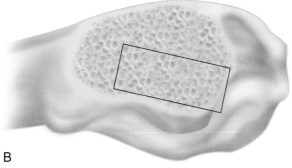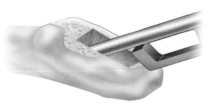

FIGURE 5 B

PEARLS

• *With cemented femoral stems, it is important to maintain a rim of cancellous bone to allow for cement interdigitation. This means not trying to fit the largest broach size possible, as in cementless implants, which would leave only cortical bone and result in a less optimal cement mantle.*

STEP 4: BROACHING

- Femoral broaches are then sequentially inserted, being sure to apply constant pressure posteriorly and laterally to avoid stem malalignment (Fig. 6A and 6B). Care should be taken to control the desired amount of version with each successive broach inserted.
- Preservation of at least 3 mm of cancellous bone medially and anteriorly is recommended (Fig. 7). If there is little remaining cancellous bone, downsize the femoral component.
- After the final broach is placed, the broach handle is removed and a trial reduction is performed. When stability and limb length have been properly restored, the hip is dislocated and the version of the stem is marked on the medial femoral neck with electrocautery or a marker. Trial components are then removed.

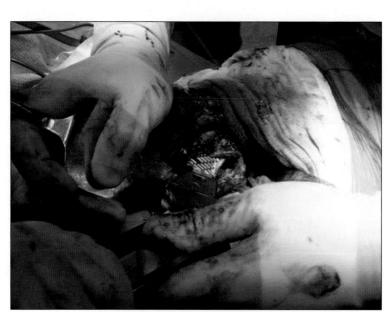

FIGURE 6   A   B

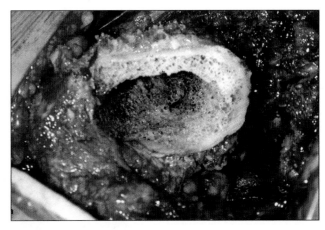

FIGURE 7

PEARLS

- *Have several sizes of cement restrictor plugs available. Attempting to insert a plug that is too large may result in fracture of the femur. If necessary, radial slits may be made in the outer plastic rings to decrease the hoop stresses created when inserting the plug.*

- *The most important factor in obtaining good cement interdigitation with the remaining cancellous bone is proper cleansing. Carefully performed pulsatile lavage is the key to obtaining this result.*

STEP 5: FINAL PREPARATION OF THE MEDULLARY CANAL

- A femoral brush is used to remove any debris or loose pieces of cancellous bone.
- Selection of a cement restrictor is based on the size of the femoral canal (Fig. 8A and 8B). Sounds included in the instrumentation may be used to determine canal diameter and the size of the distal stem centralizer. The cement plug should be at least 2 mm larger than the largest sound that passes and

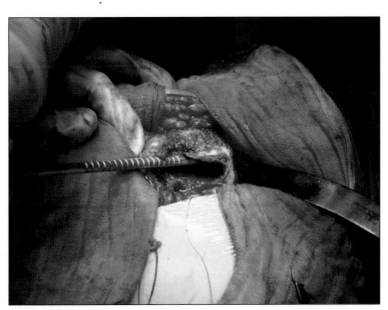
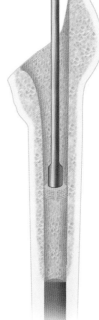

A

B

FIGURE 8

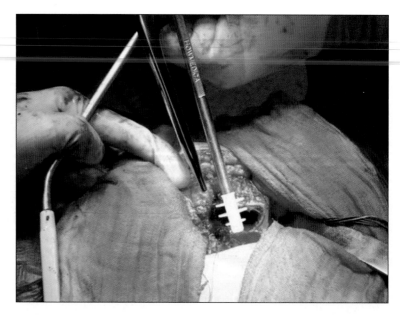

FIGURE 9

is placed approximately 1.5–2 cm distal to the tip of the femoral stem (Fig. 9).

- The proximal femoral bone is then thoroughly cleansed with a pulsatile lavage system with a long nozzle, spraying perpendicular to the long axis of the femur (Fig. 10A and 10B). The remaining cancellous

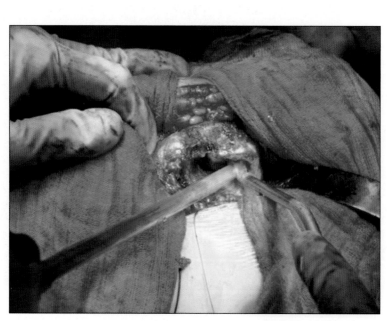

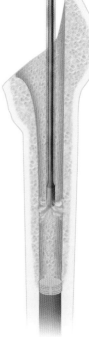

FIGURE 10   A   B

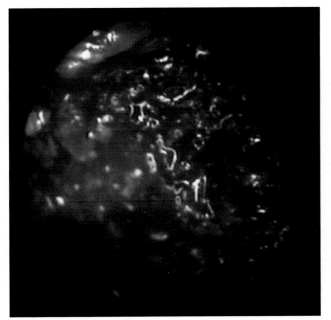

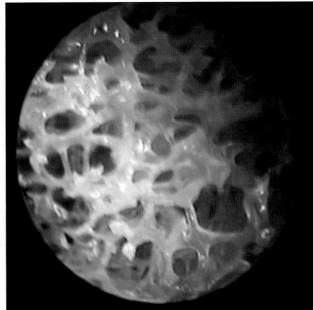

A   B

FIGURE 11

bone is irrigated until no blood or marrow tissue remains, which facilitates cement interdigitation and subsequent pressurization of the cement mantle (Fig. 11A and 11B).
- After a thorough lavage, the canal is suctioned completely dry, and the cement prepared in step 6 is immediately introduced.

STEP 6: CEMENT MIXING
- The surgeon and the operating room team should be familiar with the behavioral characteristics of the cement being used as well as with the equipment used to prepare the cement.
- Cement is mixed in a container under vacuum or with a centrifuge. Typically, two 40-mg packages of cement are mixed for a femoral stem. Occasionally patients with extremely wide "stovepipe" femurs will require three to four packages of cement to fill the canal.
- In patients with prior sepsis or with diabetes mellitus, or patients on chronic steroid therapy, consider using antibiotic-impregnated cement.

STEP 7: CEMENT APPLICATION
- Cement behavior is dependent on the room temperature and humidity, as well as the type of cement and any additives.

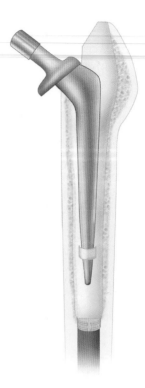

FIGURE 12

- In general, a medium-viscosity cement is preferred. When the cement delivered from the nozzle tip has lost its sheen and does not stick to the surgeon's glove, it is ready for application.
- The cement is delivered in a retrograde manner, starting just above the cement restrictor (Fig. 12). Care is taken not to bury the nozzle tip within the advancing cement, as this can create voids in the mantle.
- After filling the femur, the cement is pressurized by applying the proximal femoral seal and continuing to deploy cement. Cement is delivered in a slow, steady manner over 2–3 minutes. Appropriate pressurization is evidenced by cement extrusion from the exposed proximal femoral cortex and a complete lack of back-bleeding.

STEP 8: FEMORAL STEM INSERTION

- Selection of a femoral stem implant should be based on surgeon's preference, a review of the literature, and stem availability.
- To prevent stem malalignment and cement mantle defects, the same posterolateral starting point used for opening the femoral canal is used for stem insertion.
- The stem is slowly inserted using a stem inserter. The inserter should not be rigidly attached to the stem, but should allow for controlling stem version.

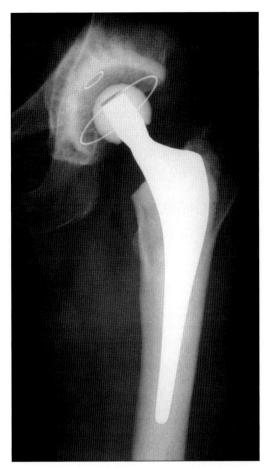

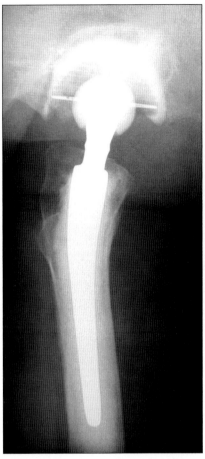

FIGURE 13   A   B

■ Cement should generally be of medium viscosity during stem insertion. Larger stems should be inserted early as they displace a larger volume of bone cement.

■ Figure 13 shows the final appearance of the femoral stem in AP (Fig. 13A) and lateral (Fig. 13B) radiographs.

Postoperative Care and Expected Outcomes

■ Patients are typically allowed to get out of bed and weight bear as tolerated on the day after surgery. For the first 4 weeks after surgery, patients use a walker or crutches and then graduate to a cane until their balance and strength have recovered.

■ Pain control begins in the operating room, with infiltration of soft tissues with local anesthetic prior to closure. Patients are routinely given patient-controlled analgesia pumps overnight after surgery and started on oral narcotic agents on postoperative day 1 if they are tolerating an oral diet.

- Every patient receives some form of deep venous thrombosis prophylaxis. Low-molecular-weight heparin products are most commonly used and are begun approximately 8 hours after surgery and then dosed daily for 2 weeks. Patients wear T.E.D. hose and pneumoboots while in bed and in the hospital.
- Physiotherapy is begun on the day after surgery and focuses on early mobilization and precautions specific to the surgical approach.

Evidence

Barrack RL, Mulroy RD, Harris WH. Improved cementing techniques and femoral component loosening in young patients with hip arthroplasty: a 12 year radiographic review. J Bone Joint Surg [Br]. 1992;74:385–9.

The authors reviewed their series of cemented femoral stems in patients younger than 50 years of age using second-generation cementing techniques, including a distal cement plug, retrograde cement delivery, and an irrigated femoral canal. Results at 12 years demonstrated that no stem had been revised for aseptic loosening, and only one stem was loose radiographically.

Majkowski RS, Miles AW, Bannister GC, Perkins T, Taylor GJS. Bone surface preparation in cemented joint replacement. J Bone Joint Surg [Br]. 1993;75:459–63.

In this study using bovine cadaver femora, the effect of nine different techniques for preparing the femur were compared with regard to cement penetration and shear strength at the cement-bone interface. The use of pressurized lavage either in a continuous or pulsed mode resulted in the greatest final cement penetration and shear strength.

McKaskie AW, Barnes MR, Lin E, Harper WM, Gregg PJ. Cement pressurization during hip replacement. J Bone Joint Surg [Br]. 1997;79:379–84.

Cement pressurization using finger-packing or a cement gun was compared in both clinical and laboratory models in this study. Cement delivery using a gun consistently produced greater maximum cement pressurization in both models. Insertion of the femoral stem produced greater pressurization than either delivery method.

Rasquinha VJ, Ranawat CS, Dua V, Ranawat AS, Rodriguez JA. A prospective, randomized, double-blind study of smooth versus rough stems using cement fixation. J Arthroplasty. 2004;19(7):2–9.

This randomized, clinical trial compared one surgeon's intermediate-term results using either rough (Ra-170) or smooth (Ra-17) stems. At a minimum of 5 years, there were no reported differences in clinical or radiographic outcomes.

Settecerri JJ, Kelley SS, Rand JA, Fitzgerald RH. Collar versus collarless cemented HD-I femoral prostheses. Clin Orthop Relat Res. 2002;(398):146–52.

In this study, 84 patients were randomized to receive either a collared or collarless femoral stem. Among the 43 patients available for follow-up at an average of 9.6 years after surgery, there were no significant differences between the groups with respect to pain, Harris Hip Score, or implant survival.

Cementless Acetabular Cup Technique

Michael D. Ries

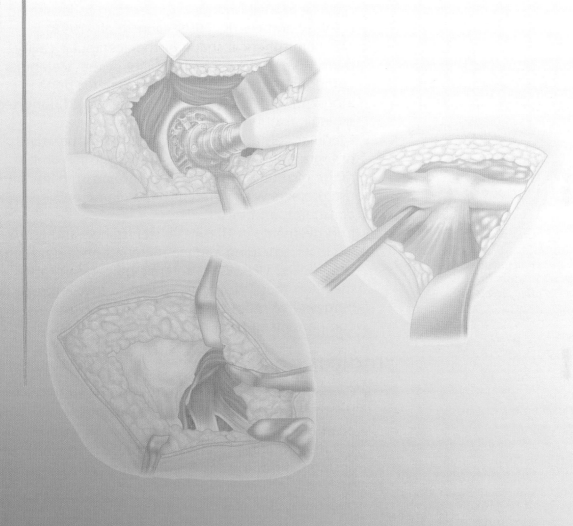

Introduction

- Use of cementless fixation in total hip arthroplasty permits direct osteointegration of the implant with long-term biologic fixation to bone.
- Problems with modular cementless acetabular components have been related to wear or mechanical failure of ultrahigh-molecular-weight polyethylene (UHMWPE) components sterilized by gamma irradiation in air, rather than to loosening (Clohisy and Harris, 1999; Dorr et al., 1998).
- The hemispherical shape of the acetabular cavity permits very good initial stability of the acetabular component and a large surface area for bone ingrowth. Once initial stability is achieved, long-term biologic fixation occurs reliably.
- Modular components also permit intraoperative optimization in implant positioning to maximize range of motion to impingement and stability, and use of liners with different head diameters, constraint, and offset.
- Improvements in UHMWPE sterilization and in alternative bearing surface materials, including highly cross-linked UHMWPE, ceramic-on-ceramic, and metal-on-metal bearings, should further improve the longevity of modular cementless acetabular components in total hip arthroplasty.

PITFALLS

- *Initial stability of an uncemented acetabular component can be achieved with use of screws, spikes, peripheral fins, or a press-fit in which the diameter of the acetabular cup is slightly larger than the reamed acetabulum. Press-fitting requires adequate acetabular bone stock. If bone stock is poor, use of a cementless acetabular component is still appropriate, but additional screw fixation is often necessary.*

Controversies

- Poor vascularity of the periarticular bone associated with radiation osteonecrosis of the pelvis may be considered a relative contraindication to cementless fixation, although cement fixation has not been associated with favorable results in this patient population either. Porous ingrowth surfaces, which provide greater initial friction between the implant and bone, may provide more reliable results with cementless fixation (Rose et al., 2006).
- Cement fixation has been advocated for use in Paget's disease, although very good results have been achieved with cementless acetabular components (Hozack et al., 1999).

Indications

- Cementless acetabular cups are indicated for treatment of symptomatic osteoarthritis, posttraumatic arthritis, or inflammatory arthritis of the hip requiring total hip arthroplasty in which the acetabular bone stock is sufficient to provide mechanical support for initial stability of an uncemented acetabular component.

Examination/Imaging

- Acetabular anatomy is best visualized on the anteroposterior pelvic radiograph. Figure 1A shows an arthritic hip in a 74-year-old man with retained hardware in the femoral head. The outline of the teardrop and acetabular joint surface is illustrated in Figure 1B. Figure 2 illustrates the amount of lateralization of the femoral head from the floor of the acetabulum. The left arrow shows the lateral border of the teardrop, which represents the anatomic floor of the acetabulum, and the right arrow represents the lateralized base of the arthritic acetabulum.

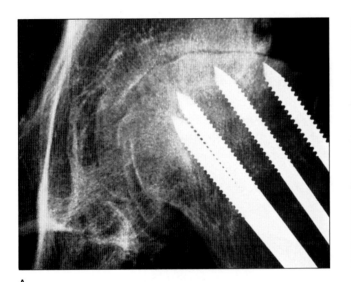
A

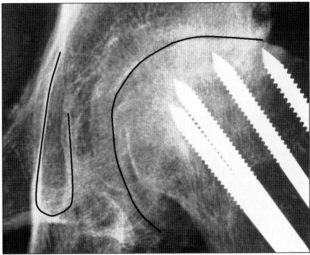
B

FIGURE 1

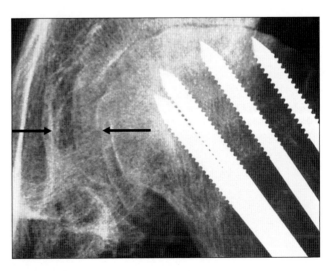

FIGURE 2

Treatment Options

- Treatment options include press-fit fixation, screw fixation, and supplemental spikes or fins.
- Press-fit fixation with a cup that is slightly larger than the reamed acetabular cavity requires both adequate peripheral coverage of the acetabular component rim and adequate bone quality. Figure 4 shows arrows that indicate that pressure from the bone against the peripheral rim of the acetabular component produces a force vector that helps to stabilize the implant while pressure against the more medial portions of the cup provides less stability.
- If the bony rim is deficient, such as that which typically occurs in dysplasia, or the bone is osteoporotic, then additional screw fixation is likely to be necessary.
- Acetabular components with supplemental spike or fin fixation do not require press-fitting or use of screws, but if the bone is sclerotic, then full seating of the acetabular component such as that shown in Figure 5 (note *arrows*) may not be possible if the spikes or fins do not fully penetrate into the hard bone.

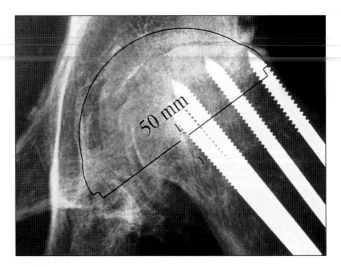

FIGURE 3

- Figure 3 shows an overlay template of the acetabular component, which is medialized to the acetabular floor and placed at 40–45° of abduction. If there is adequate lateral bone coverage of the acetabular component, as shown in this case, then peripheral coverage of the rim should be sufficient to permit press-fit stability.

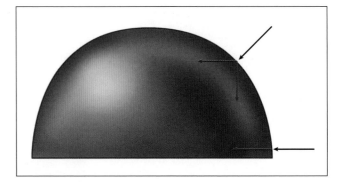

FIGURE 4

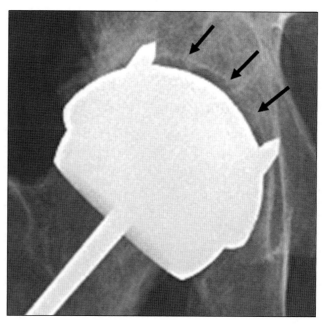

FIGURE 5

Surgical Anatomy

- Figure 6A shows the floor of the acetabulum, which is a reliable anatomic landmark and should be identified prior to reaming. The inner circular line in Figure 6B outlines the acetabular floor, and the acetabular rim is shown by the outer circular line. The acetabular floor may be covered with soft tissue or osteophytes. This represents the lateral border of the teardrop seen radiographically.

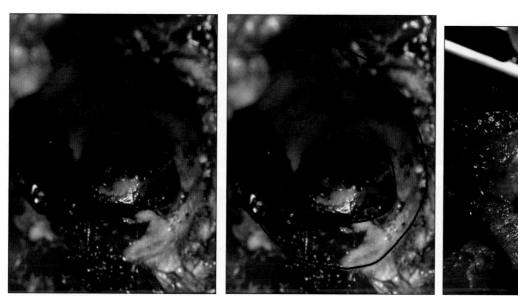

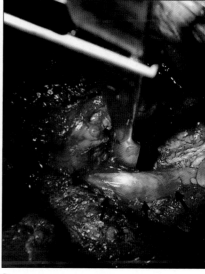

A   B   C

FIGURE 6

- The acetabular labrum should be débrided and the bony rim identified circumferentially.
- The sciatic nerve is posterior to the piriformis tendon and traverses over the surface of the ischium. It should be identified by palpation and protected during placement of acetabular retractors. The nerve is under tension during hip flexion. The hip should not be fully flexed during acetabular reaming because the posterior retractor is adjacent to the sciatic nerve and may cause nerve compression (Satcher et al., 2003). Figure 6C shows that the sciatic nerve (*arrows*) can be in close proximity to the posterior acetabular retractor when the hip is flexed.

Positioning

- For either a posterior or direct lateral (Hardinge) approach, the patient is positioned in the lateral decibitus position.

PEARLS

- *An axillary roll should be placed to protect the contralateral brachial plexus.*

- *The fibular head of the contralateral knee should be padded to prevent peroneal nerve compression.*

- *The contralateral hip should be flexed slightly since a flexion contracture could affect pelvic position.*

- *The ipsilateral arm should be placed on an upper armboard (Fig. 7A) or pillows so that it is parallel to the lower arm to avoid rotation of the upper spine.*

PITFALLS

- *No positioning device will hold the pelvis in a completely rigid position during surgery. Pelvic position should be checked periodically during the procedure by palpation of the anterior superior iliac spine (ASIS). Pelvic stability is reduced more in obese patients.*

- *If a posterior approach is used, the femur and lower leg are retracted anteriorly during acetabular preparation. The weight of the thigh and lower leg can cause the ilium to tilt forward, which may lead to insufficient anteversion of the acetabular component. Either the pelvic position should be re-established during acetabular cup placement by pulling the ilium posteriorly or the acetabular insertion device flexed to compensate for anterior tilt of the ilium.*

Equipment

- An inflatable beanbag with or without additional side supports or various devices with vertical padded posts can be used to secure the patient in the lateral decubitis position. Figure 7B shows a patient positioned using a padded post against the sacrum. Two other padded posts are placed against the pubic symphysis and ASIS to secure the patient in the lateral decubitis position. For very obese patients, it may be necessary to tape the thorax to the operating room table in order to provide more support.

Controversies

- Vertical padded post devices place pressure over bony prominences, including the pubic symphysis, ASIS, and sacrum. This provides more stability than an inflatable beanbag, but pressure over the ASIS can occasionally cause sensory disturbances in the lateral femoral cutaneous nerve (Kitson and Ashworth, 2002).

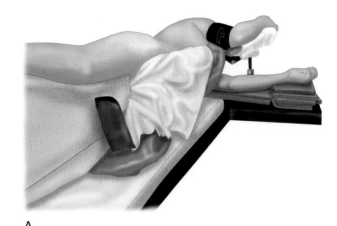

A

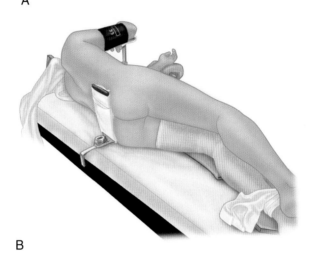

B

FIGURE 7

Instrumentation

- A self-retaining, Charnley-type retractor is used to retract the skin, subcutaneous tissue, and fascial layers. Figure 8A shows Holman or similar retractors that have been placed over the anterior and posteroinferior acetabular rims to lever the proximal femur and soft tissues. The Charnley (C), posterior Holman (P), and anterior Holman (A) retractors, and proximal femur (F) are labeled in Figure 8B.

Controversies

- Minimally invasive approaches, which retain more of the capsule and short external rotator tendon attachments to the proximal femur, may permit better hip stability and earlier return of function after surgery. However, these approaches may not be suitable in heavy patients or those with stiff hips, in whom more soft tissue dissection is needed to mobilize the femur and permit adequate acetabular exposure.

Portals/Exposures

- The hip can be exposed through a posterior, direct lateral (Hardinge), or anterior approach.

PEARLS

- *The acetabulum should be exposed circumferentially.*

- *The acetabular labrum is débrided to identify the bony rim.*

- *For a posterior approach, the femur is retracted anteriorly, and for lateral or anterior approaches, the femur is retracted posteriorly.*

PITFALLS

- *Adequate mobilization of the proximal femur is necessary to expose the acetabulum.*

- *The inferior hip capsule may restrict adequate mobilization of the femur.*

- *Circumferential capsulotomy or capsulectomy will provide better mobilization of the femur and acetabular exposure.*

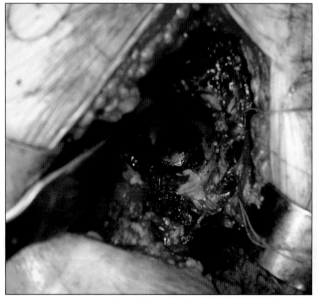

A

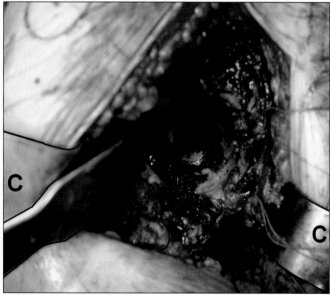

B

FIGURE 8

Instrumentation/ Implantation

• Hemispherical "cheese grater" reamers are typically used to prepare the acetabulum. Smaller "cutout" reamers may be easier to insert through small incisions but also can catch on the edge of the acetabular rim during reaming.
• A trial shell that is the same diameter as the largest reamer used should be inserted to confirm that the reamed acetabular cavity is hemispherical and the same diameter as the final reamer size.

Procedure

STEP 1: ACETABULAR REAMING

■ After the medial floor of the acetabulum is identified, a relatively small reamer is used to ream medially to the level of the acetabular floor. Figure 9 shows that the acetabular floor is in continuity with the reamed acetabulum after medialization. The reamed cavity will act to centralize successive reamers that are used to expand the acetabulum.

■ Sequential reamers, usually in 2-mm increments, are used to expand the size of the reamed acetabulum to the peripheral rim, while maintaining the integrity of the medial and lateral acetabular walls. Figure 10 shows that the floor is still seen and the acetabular walls are preserved after final reaming.

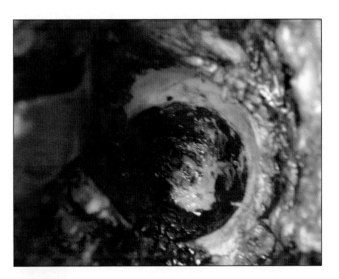

FIGURE 9

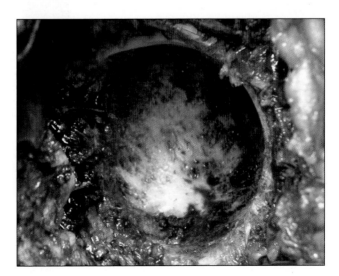

FIGURE 10

Controversies

- Medialization to the acetabular floor may not always be necessary. Medialization permits better peripheral coverage of the acetabular component, but also removes more bone than incomplete medialization. Positioning the cup in a more lateral location retains more medial bone, which may be beneficial if later cup removal and revision are needed. However, lateral placement of the center of the hip also increases joint reactive forces, which may contribute to increased wear of the bearing surface.

STEP 2: ALIGNMENT

- The acetabular component should be oriented at approximately 40–45° of abduction and 20–25° of anteversion in order to maximize stability and range of motion to impingement.
- Once the acetabular cup is inserted, a trial liner should be used. After the femoral component is inserted, range of motion to impingement and stability are assessed. If impingement occurs, then the cup position should be changed if necessary.

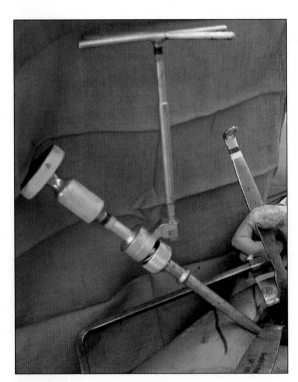

A

FIGURE 11

PEARLS

- *Mechanical alignment devices are helpful to orient the acetabular component. The vertical limb of most alignment devices is oriented at 45°, so this should be slightly more abducted than a vertical position to provide 40° of abduction (Fig. 11A). The horizontal limb of the alignment device, shown as an X-shaped bar in Figure 11B, is oriented in line with the axis of the upper body to orient the component in 20–25° of anteversion.*

PITFALLS

- *The pelvis may tilt forward during acetabular preparation and cup insertion. Pelvic position should be corrected or the acetabular cup flexed forward during insertion to compensate for any forward tilt of the ilium.*

Instrumentation

- Alignment devices usually contain a vertical positioning bar at 45° of abduction and also an anteversion guide. However, the position of the insertion device rod alone can be used and its position also assessed during cup placement.

Controversies

• Compared to mechanical alignment devices, computer templating permits more accurate acetabular cup placement, but requires additional surgical time, equipment, and staff and surgeon training. The relative benefit of computer templating may not outweigh the expense and the exposure of the patient to additional surgical time. However, further developments in computer templating with less costly and time-consuming techniques may permit more routine use of this technology.

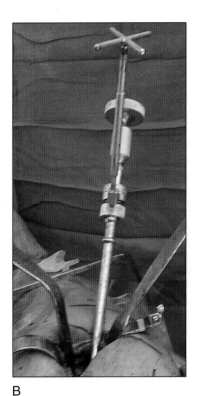

B

FIGURE 11, cont'd

• *If a constant amount of acetabular cup oversizing is selected, such as 2 mm for all acetabuli, the relative percent expansion of the acetabulum that occurs during insertion of the cup will be greater in a small compared to a large acetabulum (Ries and Harbaugh, 1997). This results in a greater risk of fracture in a small compared to a large acetabulum unless a smaller amount of oversizing is used (1 mm in small acetabuli and 2 mm in larger acetabuli).*

Instrumentation/ Implantation

• The acetabular cup should be aligned in the desired position of abduction and anteversion prior to impacting and final seating of the cup. If a change in cup position is needed, the implant should be removed completely and reoriented prior to reseating.

STEP 3: INSERTION OF A PRESS-FIT ACETABULAR COMPONENT

■ For press-fit fixation, the acetabular component is slightly larger than the reamed acetabular cavity.

■ Stability of the acetabular component is achieved from pressure of the peripheral acetabular bone against the rim of the component, while pressure against the more medial portions of the cup produces a force vector against the cup, which tends to provide less stability (see Fig. 4).

■ After insertion of the metal shell, peripheral osteophytes (*arrows* in Fig. 12A) are removed with an osteotome or rongeur to prevent impingement.

■ Figure 12B shows the postoperative position of a press-fit acetabular cup. The acetabular component has been medialized to the teardrop or acetabular floor, and there is adequate lateral coverage to permit stable press-fit stability.

Controversies

• Press-fit fixation avoids use of screws or cups with screw holes, but also results in a risk of acetabular fracture or inadequate fixation. Excellent clinical results have been achieved with cups having screws, so the need for press-fit fixation is not clear. However, use of an implant without screw holes provides a large surface area for support of the liner, limits access of debris through screw holes, and is necessary for large-diameter metal-on-metal resurfacing arthroplasty.

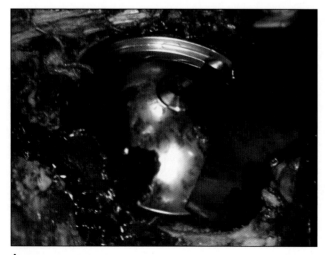

A

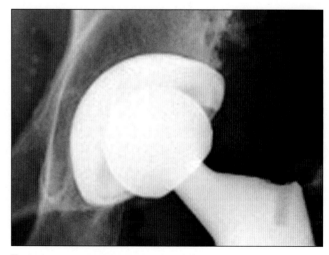

B

FIGURE 12

Instrumentation/ Implantation

• Flexible drill bits and screwdrivers are necessary to insert screws through the dome of the acetabular cup. Both the drill and screwdriver should be inserted with the handle as horizontal as possible to maximize torque during insertion. The distal end of the incision limits how horizontal the drill or screwdriver can be placed.

Controversies

• Screw fixation can be achieved with either dome or peripheral screws. Peripheral screws require a cup with a large enough metallic rim to provide circumferential metal around the screw head, which can limit the inner diameter of the cup and size of the liner used.

STEP 4: SCREW FIXATION

■ Figure 13A shows a long (40- to 50-mm) intramedullary iliac screw, which has been placed superiorly and does not exit through the cortex of the ilium. A short (20- to 25-mm) screw has been placed posteriorly toward the sciatic notch, which exits through the outer table of the pelvis.

■ The most commonly used cup sizes include two rings of screw holes, such as those shown in Figure 13B. The long superior iliac screw is placed through a screw hole in the inner ring while the posterior screw may be inserted through either the inner or outer ring screw holes (Fig. 13C and 13D).

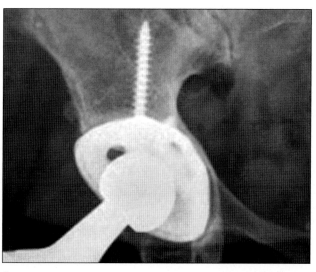

A

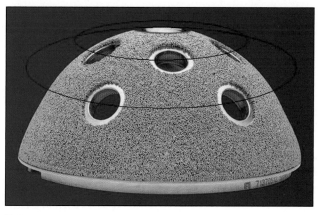

B

FIGURE 13

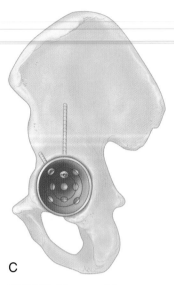

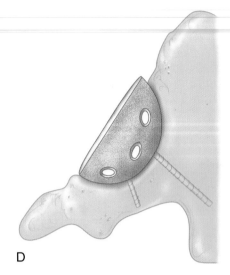

C   D

FIGURE 13, cont'd

PEARLS

- *If postoperative radiation therapy is required to minimize the risk of heterotopic bone formation, the acetabular component bone-implant interface should be shielded to permit bone ingrowth into the surface of the component.*

PITFALLS

- *An anteroposterior radiograph should be obtained in the recovery room after surgery to ensure adequate reduction of the hip and component placement.*

- *Dislocation may occur while the patient is under anesthesia, during transfers, or during positioning in the recovery room, particularly if long-acting spinal anesthetics are used, which result in decreased muscle tone.*

Controversies

- Weight-bearing stresses can cause torque on the acetabular component, which could lead to early displacement, particularly with a press-fit technique in relatively poor bone stock. However, displacement of an acetabular component in the early postoperative period likely requires trauma such as would occur from a fall. Even with full weight-bearing activity permitted, use of some type of ambulatory support (walker or crutches) is appropriate to minimize the risk of a postoperative fall.

Postoperative Care and Expected Outcomes

- Hip dislocation precautions should be followed.
- Weight bearing does not necessarily need to be restricted. Weight-bearing restriction is typically required for use of an uncemented femoral component, which can subside, but the acetabular component is inherently stable because of the hemispherical geometry of the acetabular cavity, and can tolerate early weight-bearing stresses.

Evidence

Clohisy JC, Harris WH. The Harris-Galante porous-coated acetabular component with screw fixation: an average ten-year follow-up study. J Bone Joint Surg [Am]. 1999;81:66–73.

One hundred seventy-seven patients (196 hips) with cementless porous coated Harris Galante acetabular components were reviewed after an average follow-up of 122 months. Eight well fixed acetabular shells (4 percent) were revised: three were revised because of dissociation of the liner, three were revised during revision of the femoral component, and two were revised because of retroacetabular osteolysis. No acetabular component migrated, was radiographically loose, or was revised because of aseptic loosening.

Dorr LD, Wan Z, Cohen J. Hemispheric titanium porous coated acetabular component without screw fixation. Clin Orthop Relat Res. 1998;(351):158–68.

One hundred eight patients (115 hips) with cementless anatomic porous replacement hemispheric acetabular components implanted without screw fixation were evaluated after an average follow-up of 6 years. No acetabular metal shell had been revised for loosening or was radiographically loose. Reoperation was required in nine (8 percent) hips because of polyethylene insert wear or dissociation.

Hozack WJ, Rushton SA, Carey C, Sakalkale D, Rothman RH. Uncemented total hip arthroplasty in Pagets disease of the hip. J Arthroplasty. 1999;14:872–6.

Five patients with Paget's disease involving the acetabulum were treated with cementless acetabular components during total hip arthroplasty. At an average follow-up of 5.8 years, all acetabular components were well fixed radiographically with no migration or loosening.

Kitson J, Ashworth MJ: Meralgia paraesthetica: a complication of patient positioning device in total hip replacement. J Bone Joint Surg [Br]. 2002;84:589–90.

The authors described three patients who developed meralgia paraesthetica in association with the use of padded post positioning devices during total hip arthroplasty.

Ries MD, Harbaugh M. Acetabular strains produced by oversized press fit cups. Clin Orthop Relat Res. 1997;(334):276–81.

Using finite element analysis, the authors found that with a constant amount of oversizing (for example, a cup which is one mm larger than the reamed acetabulum for all acetabular sizes) the relative expansion of the acetabulum and risk of fracture during press fitting will be greater in a small compared to a large acetabulum.

Rose PS, Halasy M, Hanssen AD, Sim FH, Lewallen DG, Berry DJ. Total Hip Arthroplasty After Pelvic Radiation: Results with Trabecular Metal Acetabular Components. Washington, DC: American Academy of Orthopedic Surgeons, 2006.

Twelve patients (13 hips) with previous pelvic irradiation therapy were treated with cementless acetabular reconstruction using trabecular metal components. After an average follow-up of 29 months none of the components had migrated or loosened.

Satcher R, Noss RS, Yingling C, Ressler J, Ries MD. The use of motor evoked potentials to monitor sciatic nerve status during revision total hip arthroplasty. J Arthroplasty. 2003;18:329–32.

Motor-evoked potentials (MEPs) were used in combination with electromyography (EMG) monitoring during revision total hip arthroplasty in 27 patients. Significant electrical events occurred, most commonly during acetabular retraction while the hip was in a flexed position.

Cementless Femoral Stems

Claire F. Young and Steven J. MacDonald

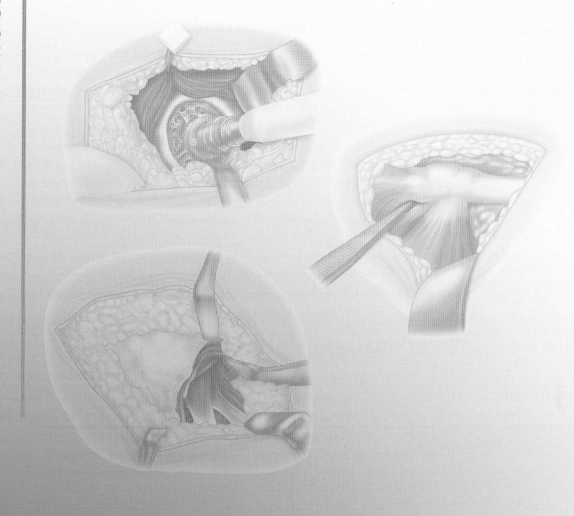

Controversies

- The best stem shape, tapered or cylindrical distal fit, remains a topic of debate. Both techniques are described.

Treatment Options

- Nonoperative measures utilizing a combination of analgesics, nonsteroidal anti-inflammatory drugs, walking aids, and activity modification to control the patient's symptomatology are effective in early stages of the disease.
- Other techniques for implanting modular uncemented stems or cemented prostheses, or for resurfacing arthroplasty, are available in addition to the cementless stem described here.

Indications

- Symptomatic arthritis in patients who have failed conservative measures.
- Patients should have suitable proximal femoral morphology for implantation of an uncemented stem, champagne flute shaped and funnel shaped.

Examination/Imaging

- A standard hip examination, including assessment of preoperative limb length discrepancy, should be done. Assessing the patient's perception of any limb length discrepancy is essential.
- Plain radiographs:
  - Anteroposterior (AP) radiograph of the pelvis, AP and lateral radiographs of the hip (Fig. 1A and 1B).
  - Proximal femoral morphology can be evaluated to assess suitability for implantation of uncemented stem (Fig. 2). As seen in Figure 2, Dorr type A and type B femoral canals are suitable for uncemented fixation, whereas type C may be more challenging. Appropriate templating should be performed for the implant chosen. This has been described in Procedure 4.

Surgical Anatomy

- The greater trochanter lies slightly posterior and lateral to the axis of the femur. The gluteus medius tendon attaches to the lateral border and minimus tendon anteriorly.
- The piriformis tendon attaches to a fossa on the medial aspect of the greater trochanter—this is the landmark for accessing the femoral canal.
- The sciatic nerve leaves the pelvis through the greater sciatic foramen, below the piriformis, and traverses the thigh in the posterior aspect. Care must be taken when placing retractors behind the trochanter, to elevate the proximal femur in the wound, that the nerve is protected.

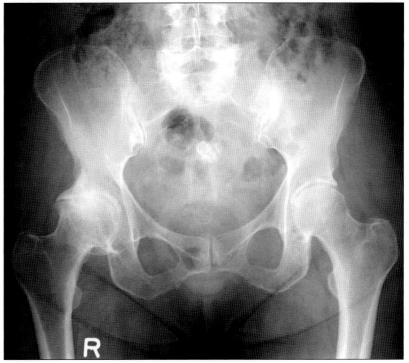

A

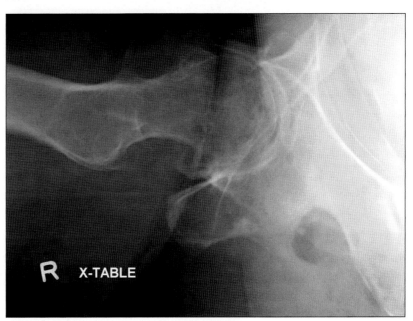

FIGURE 1   B

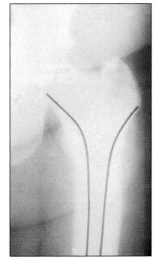

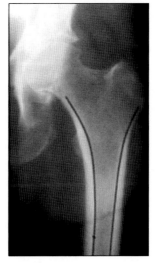

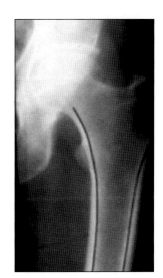

FIGURE 2   A   B   C

Equipment

• Anterior and posterior positioning bolsters

Controversies

• Patients can be placed supine on the table for the procedure.

Positioning

■ Lateral positioning of the patient is used, with the affected side uppermost and the pelvis fixed with anterior and posterior bolsters.
■ The limb is draped free, and a "dislocation bag" is attached to the drapes to keep the foot sterile.
■ The femur should be rotated internally (posterior approach) or externally (lateral approach) so that the tibia is perpendicular to the floor and the proximal femur is delivered into the wound (Fig. 3).

Portals/Exposures

■ Exposures for total hip arthroplasty have been described in Procedures 5 and 6.

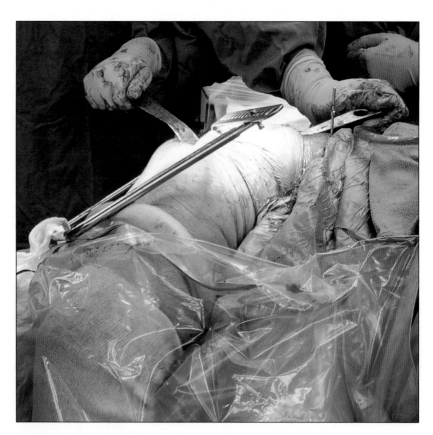

FIGURE 3

Instrumentation/Implantation

- A limb length and offset guide and appropriate pin may be used for accurate measurement.
- A power saw is used to make the femoral neck osteotomy.

Procedure

STEP 1

- During the exposure and prior to dislocation of the hip, the limb length and offset are assessed using a leg length/offset guide. The hip is positioned so that the knees and feet of both limbs are aligned.
- A transverse mark is made with diathermy and a marking pen on the highest point of the greater trochanter.
- A short pin with a guide stop is then inserted into the iliac wing through a small stab incision.
- The limb length and offset guide is then set for the patient's preoperative leg length and hip offset (Fig. 4). The guide is then placed on the back table and not adjusted; it will be required for assessing the limb length and offset after reconstruction of the joint.
- The femoral neck should be osteotomized at the appropriate level as determined by preoperative templating for the prosthesis to be implanted (normally a finger breadth above the level of the lesser trochanter).

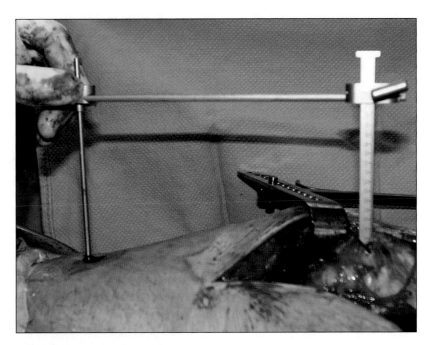

FIGURE 4

Controversies

- Leg length can also be assessed by placing both feet together and assessing the relative position of the knees, although this is less accurate than using a guide. The relative abduction/adduction positions of the legs must be taken into account if using this method.
- Various designs of stems are available, such as tapered, cylindrical, and anatomic. Step 1 is the same for all. Tapered and cylindrical stem femoral preparation and implantation are discussed separately below.
  - The tapered stem type is designed with a proximal-to-distal taper to wedge into the metaphyseal region of the femur. The proximal part of the stem has a porous coat to enhance initial stability and allow for bone ingrowth. The geometric design of this stem means it can subside into a position of maximal fit, which improves load sharing of the device with proximal bone.
  - The cylindrical stem gains initial stability with tight diaphyseal fit. The canal is machined to accommodate the stem, which maximizes its potential for bone ingrowth by being fully porous coated.

PEARLS

- *Clearing the soft tissue from the piriformis fossa aids in establishing the correct entry point for the box osteotome, ensuring that this is lateralized appropriately.*

- *Placing blunt retractors around the femoral shaft at the level of the calcar can help to "gunsight" a straight passage down the canal.*

PITFALLS

- *Care must be taken to stay lateral with the box osteotome to ensure that subsequent reaming and broaching are in alignment with the femoral axis.*

Instrumentation/ Implantation

- A box osteotome is required to open the femoral canal.

Procedure: Tapered Stem Technique

STEP 2

- The piriformis fossa is identified and the femoral canal is opened with a box osteotome (Fig. 5). The femoral canal is opened.
- A canal finder can then be inserted down the canal to identify a straight passage down the femur (Fig. 6).

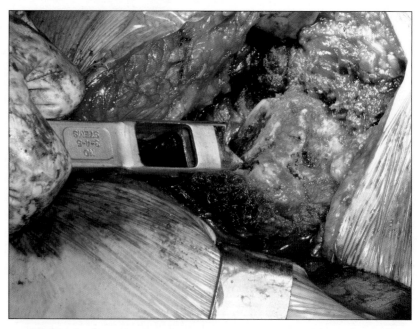

FIGURE 5

PEARLS

- *Ensure that the reamer remains lateral and in alignment with the femoral canal to ensure placement in the center of the medullary canal.*

- *Creating a groove in the medial aspect of the greater trochanter will allow axial canal reaming.*

PITFALLS

- *Varus placement of the reamer will result in undersizing of the implant.*

- *Care must be taken while using the reamer to avoid damage to the abductor muscles.*

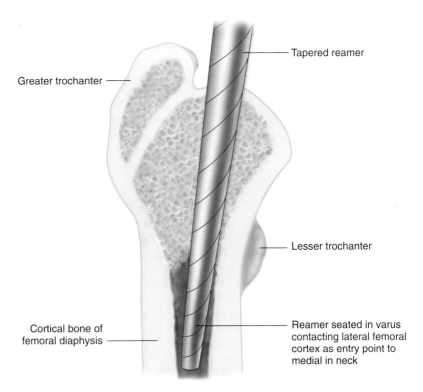

Greater trochanter

Tapered reamer

Lesser trochanter

Cortical bone of femoral diaphysis

Reamer seated in varus contacting lateral femoral cortex as entry point to medial in neck

FIGURE 6

Instrumentation/ Implantation

- Sequentially sized femoral canal reamers

STEP 3

- The smallest tapered reamer is used to begin reaming the femoral canal. Insert the reamer starting slightly posterolaterally to ensure access to the center of the medullary canal.
- Sequential reamers are then used to enlarge the canal until firm cortical reaming is felt. The depth of adequate insertion, in relation to the greater trochanter, is usually marked on the reamer (Fig. 7).

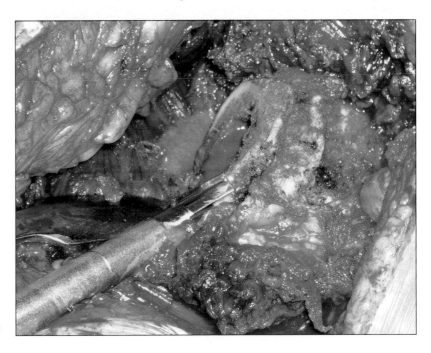

FIGURE 7

The decision regarding the final component size is based on the fit of the broach, not the reamer. Reaming should be stopped once resistance is felt to avoid using a reamer size that will be oversized relative to the final broach size.

■ If intraoperative sizing is found to be much less than templated sizing, there is a high probability that the femoral preparation is in varus.

STEP 4

■ The femoral canal is then broached to remove cancellous bone, maintaining the axis in alignment with the axis of the femur. The broach should be inserted maintaining the required anteversion of the femoral neck. An anteversion guide can be attached to the broach handle to ensure that appropriate anteversion is achieved (Fig. 8).

■ Start with a broach three sizes smaller than the largest reamer used. Insert the broach until the top reaches the level of the neck resection. Sequential broaches should be inserted until the templated size is reached. This should be seated so that the top of the broach is level with the neck resection. The selected final broach should be rotationally stable within the femoral canal, and this should be assessed by attempting to rotate the broach within the femur.

PEARLS

• *Occasionally backing the broach out of the canal a short distance before further advancement, which cleans the broach teeth of bone, allows easier advancement.*

PITFALLS

• *Care is required to maintain the broach laterally in alignment with the femoral canal to prevent varus positioning.*

• *The abductor musculature should be protected to prevent damage from the broach.*

• *Care must be taken on removing the broach to ensure that the greater trochanter is not fractured. Placing a slight varus force on the broach handle when it is being removed will help minimize the risk of fracture.*

Instrumentation/ Implantation

• Sequentially sized femoral canal broaches, a broach handle, anteversion handle, and mallet
• Calcar planar reamer

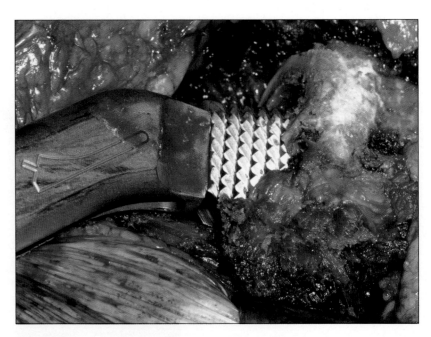

FIGURE 8

- Stability can be checked by attempting to retrovert the stem using the broach handle. Stability is indicated if there is no movement at the bone-broach interface.
- If the size of broach selected does not achieve stability in the bone, it should be removed, the next-sized reamer inserted to the appropriate depth, and then the canal broached again using the corresponding-sized broach. Stability should then be rechecked. For example, if a size 3 broach did not achieve rotational stability, remove the broach, ream with a size 4 reamer, and insert a size 4 broach before rechecking stability.
- The broach handle is removed, leaving the broach in the femoral canal, and the calcar is reamed using the planar reamer, which fits over the broach trunion.

Step 5

- A trial neck, standard or high offset as determined by templating, is placed on the broach. A trial femoral head of the chosen diameter and length is applied and the hip is reduced.
- Hip stability is then checked with the hip in full extension and external rotation, and in full flexion and internal rotation. The feet are then opposed and the limb length and offset checked with the guide that was set previously. Instability is an indication of the joint being too loose, bony impingement, or component malposition.
- The hip can be retrialed using different options of neck offset and neck length until the desired stability, offset, and limb length are achieved.

PEARLS

- *If the femoral head is equatorial in the acetabulum with the limb in 20° of flexion and 30° of internal rotation, then component position is correct.*

- *If trial placement demonstrates leg length to be perfect with the shortest available head, be wary, as the femoral component final position will normally be 2–3 mm proud from the final broach position. If trial placement demonstrates this finding, rebroach to seat the broach (and therefore the femoral implant) a few millimeters further.*

Instrumentation/ Implantation

- Offset options for different broach sizes and selection of femoral heads of required head diameter with different neck lengths

Instrumentation/Implantation

• Femoral stem introducer and mallet

STEP 6

■ The selected femoral stem is now implanted after removing the broach. The stem is attached to the stem inserter and entered into the femoral canal. Hand insertion should enable the stem to be inserted to within one finger breadth of the proximal extent of the porous coating (Fig. 9). The stem can then be seated fully by gentle mallet blows.

■ The selected trial head is then placed on the Morse taper and the hip reduced to reassess stability and limb length. The Morse taper is washed and dried and the definitive selected head is implanted.

■ The hip joint is thoroughly washed, taking care to ensure there is no debris in the acetabulum, and the hip is reduced.

■ The capsule should be sutured. The hip approach is then closed in layers.

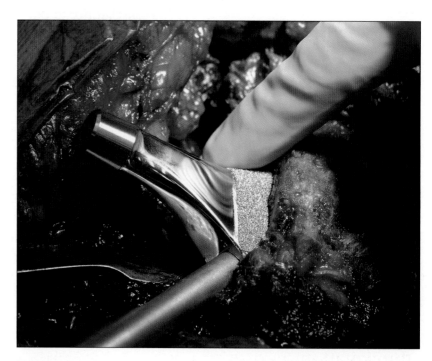

FIGURE 9

Instrumentation/ Implantation

- Pilot hole drill
- Sequentially sized intramedullary reamers

Instrumentation/ Implantation

- Femoral broaches and a mallet
- Trial necks for broach and assorted heads

Procedure: Cylindrical Stem Technique

STEP 2

- A pilot hole is placed in the piriformis fossa.
- The canal is then reamed with sequential reamers until a good bite of the endosteal cortical bone is felt. The aim is to ream the diaphyseal canal to obtain 5 cm of cortical fit with a reamer that is 0.5 mm smaller than the proposed stem size (Fig. 10).

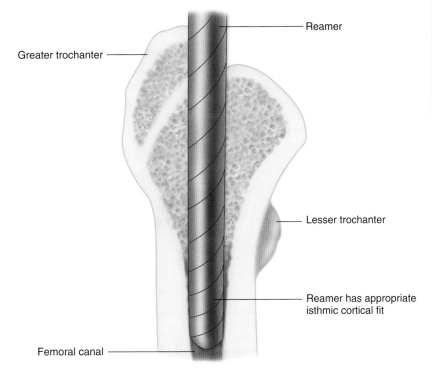

Reamer

Greater trochanter

Lesser trochanter

Reamer has appropriate isthmic cortical fit

Femoral canal

FIGURE 10

STEP 3

- Begin with the smallest broach and increase until broach size matches the component size (based on the size of the distal reaming).
- The appropriate-size broach is selected and impacted into the femoral canal, maintaining the correct anteversion, to the level of the neck cut. The rotational plane for the broach is that of the femoral neck cut.
- A trial neck and head are then applied to the broach trunion and a trial reduction of the hip is performed. Limb length and offset and hip stability are tested as for the tapered stem. Appropriate adjustments are made to ensure that the hip is stable and there is adequate restoration of limb length and offset.

STEP 4

- The chosen definitive stem is then implanted following broach removal. It should be possible to insert the stem by hand pressure to a depth requiring 5 cm advancement (to achieve diaphyseal fixation over 4–6 cm) by mallet blows on the introducer.

Controversies

- Restricting weight bearing during the first 6 weeks of rehabilitation is controversial.

Postoperative Care and Expected Outcomes

- An abduction pillow is placed between the patient's legs to prevent adduction and potential dislocation. This may be maintained while the patient is in bed for the first 6 weeks.
- Mobilization is commenced on day 1. Weight bearing may be limited to 50% for the first 6 weeks as bone ingrowth commences.
- The patient is discouraged from flexing the hip beyond 90° or hip adduction (crossing the legs) for the first 6 weeks as the soft tissues heal.
- Abductor strengthening exercises are commenced after 6 weeks.
- Following radiographs taken at 6 weeks to ensure implant stability, the patient increases to full weight bearing and is weaned off walking aids.
- Patients should anticipate return to normal activities unaided by 12 weeks.

Evidence

Bourne RB, Rorabeck CH, Patterson JJ, Guerin J. Tapered titanium cementless total hip replacements. Clin Orthop Relat Res. 2001;(393):112–20.

This study is a retrospective review of 307 total hip replacements with a tapered titanium cementless stem. It reports good survivorship of the femoral stem at minimum 10 years' follow-up. [Case series]

Chen CJ, Xenos JS, McAuley JP, Young A, Engh CA Sr. Second-generation porous coated total hip arthroplasties have high survival. Clin Orthop Relat Res. 2006;(466):66.

This retrospective review of 157 consecutive hip replacements with a fully porous-coated cylindrical femoral component reports 99% survivorship at 5 years with bone ingrowth evident in 99% of stems. [Case series]

Dorr LD, Faugere MC, Mackel AM, Gruen TA, Bognar B, Malluche HH. Structural and cellular assesssment of bone quality of proximal femur. Bone. 1993;14:231–42.

This clinical study describes radiographic measurement of proximal femoral morphology and correlates it to bone histomophometry. It describes radiographic features that are favorable for uncemented stem implantation. [Grade 1 recommendation]

Engh Jr CA, Claus AM, Hopper RH, Engh CA. Long term results using anatomic medullary locking hip prosthesis. Clin Orthop Relat Res. 2001;(393):137–46.

This study reviews 223 consecutive hips using a cylindrical femoral component with a mean 13.9-year follow-up. [Case series]

Mallory TH, Lombardi AV, Leith JR, Fujita H, Hartman JF, Capps SG, Kefawa CA, Adams JB, Vorys GC. Minimal 10-year results of a tapered cementless femoral component in total hip arthroplasty. J Arthroplasty. 2001;16(Suppl 1):49–54.

This paper reports a series of 120 hips with a dual-tapered femoral component. Results show a survivorship of 97.5% at a mean follow-up of 12.2 years. [Case series]

Hip Resurfacing Arthroplasty

Wadih Y. Matar and Paul E. Beaulé

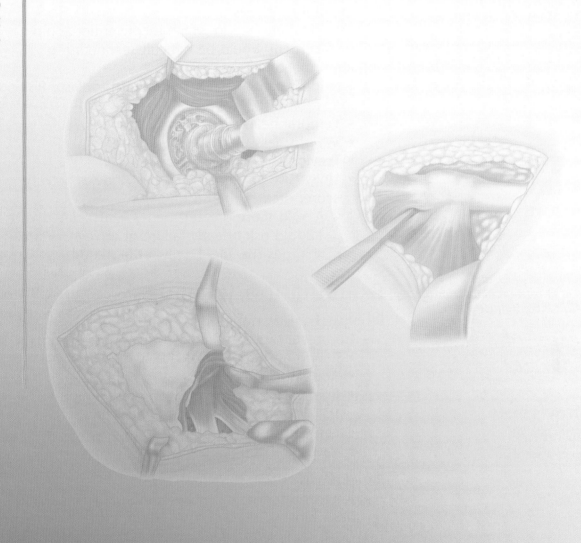

Controversies

- Women of childbearing age
- Patients older than 65 years

Indications

- Advanced osteoarthritis (OA) in the young adult (age <60 years) in whom a conventional total hip replacement (THR) may not last a lifetime, therefore requiring a revision procedure.
- Primary or secondary OA: osteonecrosis, trauma, Legg-Calvé-Perthes disease, developmental dysplasia of the hip (Crowe class I and II), or slipped capital femoral epiphysis.
- Posttraumatic hip in which a conventional hip replacement would be difficult secondary to abnormal anatomy.
- The ideal patient has a Surface Arthroplasty Risk Index (SARI) ≤3:
  - Femoral head cyst: 1 cm=2 points
  - Weight: less than 80 kg=2 points
  - Previous hip surgery: 1 point
  - University of California at Los Angeles activity score: greater than 6=1 point
    - ◆ A SARI score greater than 3 is associated with a 12-fold risk of early failure or adverse radiologic changes (Beaulé, Dorey, et al., 2004).

Examination/Imaging

PHYSICAL EXAMINATION

- Complete hip examination with emphasis on:
  - Range of motion (ROM)
  - Abductors strength
  - Impingement sign: pain on passive hip flexion to 90°, internal rotation, and adduction
  - Leg length discrepancy
  - Vascular examination

RADIOGRAPHS

- Anteroposterior (AP) pelvis radiograph, including both hips.
- Cross-table lateral radiograph of the affected hip.
- Reduced anterior femoral head-neck offset or a pistol grip deformity. Offset of Eijer less than 0.15 is abnormal (Beaulé et al., 2007).

TEMPLATING

- We use the Conserve Plus hip resurfacing prosthesis (Wright Medical Technology, Arlington, TN)
- Templating is the most important preoperative step for a successful outcome.

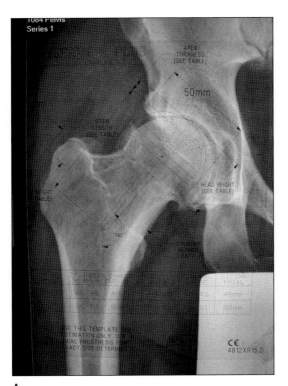

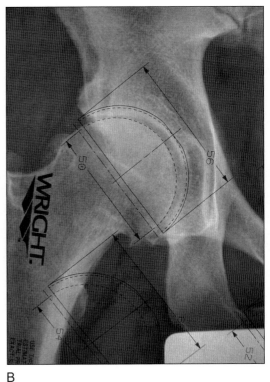

A   B

FIGURE 1

- The template, which is magnified by 15%, is placed over the AP (Fig. 1A and 1B) and lateral views:
  - Anteroposterior view
    - The femoral head is sized first. The dotted lines in Figure 1A indicate the level of reaming by the cylindrical reamer. Femoral neck notching should be avoided.
    - The acetabulum is subsequently sized, keeping in mind that the Conserve Plus shell thickness is available in two sizes, 3 and 5 mm, allowing us to deal with femoral head–to-acetabulum mismatch. For example, a femoral head that is sized to 50 mm can be matched to a 56-mm acetabular normal-thickness cup in a normal acetabulum, or a 60-mm increased-thickness cup in a shallow and widened acetabulum.

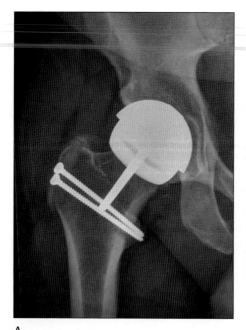
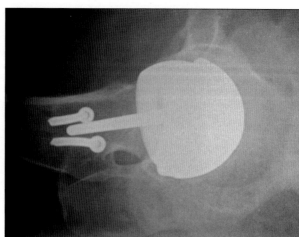

A   B

FIGURE 2

- Lateral view
  - ◆ The orientation of the femoral component is gauged on the lateral view to re-establish the anterior femoral head-to-neck offset ratio (Fig. 2A and 2B). Anterior translation may be needed to re-establish anterior offset.

COMPUTED TOMOGRAPHY
- Assesses bony architecture (osteophytes, fracture fragments)

Surgical Anatomy

- The most common surgical approach for resurfacing remains the posterior approach. The approach described in this procedure is one that uses the surgical hip dislocation approach as described by Ganz et al. (2001). The advantages of this approach over the posterior approach are less soft tissue dissection as well as preservation of the extraosseous femoral head blood supply, which may play a role in preventing femoral component loosening and femoral neck fracture.
- The femoral head blood supply is mainly derived from the medial femoral circumflex artery (MFCA), with a lesser contribution from the lateral circumflex (Fig. 3).

Treatment Options

- Nonoperative treatment.
- Hemiresurfacing can be used as a time-buying option for patients less than 30 years of age with a large osteonecrotic lesion either at the pre- or postcollapse stage with minimal acetabular cartilage involvement.
- Total hip replacement.

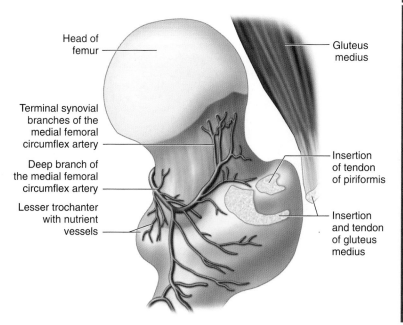

Head of femur

Gluteus medius

Terminal synovial branches of the medial femoral circumflex artery

Deep branch of the medial femoral circumflex artery

Lesser trochanter with nutrient vessels

Insertion of tendon of piriformis

Insertion and tendon of gluteus medius

FIGURE 3

- The anatomy of the MCFA is well described by Gautier et al. (2000).
- The MFCA is almost always derived from the deep femoral artery. One of its five branches, the deep branch, courses toward the intertrochanteric crest between the pectineus and the obturator externus. Posteriorly, it can found between the inferior gemellus and the quadratus femoris. It remains posterior to the tendon of the obturator externus and anterior to the tendons of the superior gemellus, obturator internus, and inferior gemellus.
- At the level of the hip capsule, it penetrates the joint just cranial to the insertion of the superior gemellus tendon and distal to the piriformis tendon. It subsequently gives off two to four retinacular branches that course beneath the synovial sheath and perforate 2–4 mm lateral to the bone-cartilage junction of the femoral head via the nutritive femoral foramina.

Positioning

- Spinal anesthetic is used for most of our hip resurfacing.
- The patient is placed in the lateral decubitus position, with the pelvis and thorax stabilized with padded bolsters.
- The entire leg is prepped and free draped. A leg cover is used up to the midthigh level.

PEARLS

- *Extending the hip facilitates the mobilization of the iliotibial band.*

- *Leaving part of the gluteus medius tendon attached to the main trochanteric fragment ensures that the osteotomy remains extracapsular.*

- *Irrigate the saw blade thoroughly to avoid overheating.*

PITFALLS

- *GT osteotomy site marking is critical in keeping the wafer viable and avoiding penetrating into the femoral neck as well as the branch of the MFCA supplying the retinacular vessels.*

- *Often the arthritic hip is fixed in external rotation, thus it may not be possible to sufficiently internally rotate the leg in order to obtain the proper plane for the osteotomy. In this situation, the surgeon must compensate for the deformity by aiming the saw blade laterally to avoid penetrating into the femoral neck.*

Portals/Exposures

- A slightly posteriorly concave incision is made centered over the greater trochanter (GT) and measuring approximately 12–14 cm (Fig. 4).
- The iliotibial band is divided from distal to proximal between the tensor and gluteus maximus. Further subcutaneous release can be performed as needed. In large men, it may be easier to split the gluteus maximus muscle.
- The trochanteric bursa is then incised.
- The gluteus maximus is retracted with a right-angle retractor to identify the posterior border of the gluteus medius as well as the junction between the gluteus minimus and the piriformis.
- With the leg in 15° of internal rotation and resting on a padded Mayo stand, the GT osteotomy is marked using cautery, leaving a 2-mm cuff of gluteus medius tendon attached to the main trochanteric fragment (Fig. 5A and 5B). The osteotomy exits proximally just lateral to the medial portion of the gluteus medius and distally past the vastus lateralis tubercule.
- The vastus lateralis is then elevated from its tubercle distally to the midlevel of the gluteus maximus insertion. Careful attention is paid so as not to compromise the vastus lateralis origin on the GT.

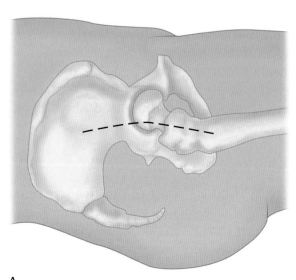

A

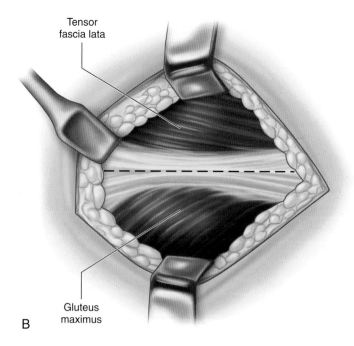

Tensor fascia lata

Gluteus maximus

B

FIGURE 4

Anterior   Posterior

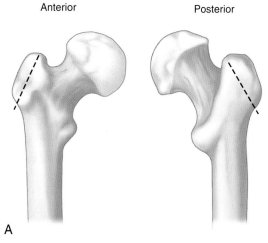

A

Fascia lata | Gluteus minimus | Gluteus medius | Piriformis | Vastus lateralis | 10-15° internal rotation

Gluteus maximus   Gamelli and obturator internus   Quadratus

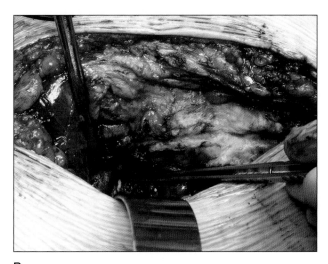

B

FIGURE 5

Instrumentation

• Blunt Hohmann retractor

Controversies

• Risk of trochanteric nonunion is 1–2% (Beaulé et al., 2007).

■ Using a 3.2-mm drill bit, the GT osteotomy wafer is predrilled in its proximal third, aiming inferomedially toward the lesser trochanter. The latter facilitates the reduction of the GT osteotomy at the end of the procedure.

■ A thin saw blade (0.09 mm) is used to perform the osteotomy.

■ A Hohmann retractor is then used to elevate the GT wafer (Fig. 6). The vastus lateralis is further elevated distally, and the remainder of the gluteus medius is released from the femur. This can be done by following the proximal edge of the piriformis tendon and retracting the gluteus minimus superoanteriorly.

■ The dissection off the anterior capsule requires a sharp dissection since the plane between the iliofemoral ligament/capsule and the gluteus minimus can be difficult to develop.

■ The leg is then placed in flexion and external rotation to allow the elevation of the vastus lateralis and intermedius from the lateral and anterior aspect of the proximal femur (Fig. 7).

■ With further flexion and elevation and the use of a right-angle retractor for the gluteus medius and minimus, the capsule is exposed. It is then incised using a Z-shaped incision along the axis of the femoral neck inferiorly and the acetabular rim posteriorly (Fig. 8). Careful attention is paid to the retinacular vessels traveling along the superior edge of the femoral neck.

■ The capsule is then elevated from the acetabular rim while avoiding the area posterior to the lesser trochanter in order to protect the main branch of the MFCA.

■ The hip is then dislocated with flexion, external rotation, and adduction of the leg using a bone hook under the femoral neck.

■ With the hip dislocated, the trochanteric wafer is folded in anteriorly and the leg is kept in flexion and external rotation in a sterile cover hanging over the edge of the operating table.

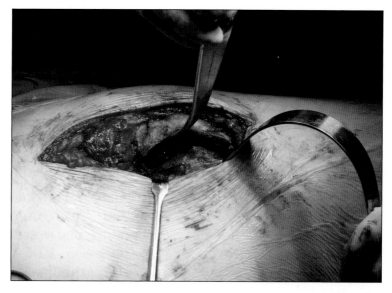

FIGURE 6

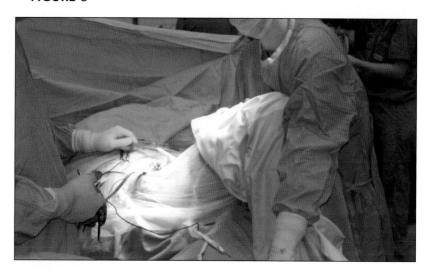

FIGURE 7

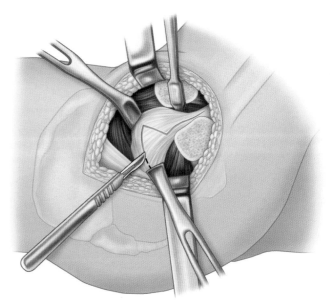

FIGURE 8

PEARLS

- *If the true head-neck junction is not properly visualized due to osteophytes, the latter can be removed with a ¾-inch curved osteotome with careful attention so as to not damage the retinacular vessels. The use of the see-through gauge facilitates proper bony removal.*

PITFALLS

- *Varus position of the femoral component is associated with a higher risk of premature failure due to loosening (Beaulé, Lee, et al., 2004).*

- *Excessive valgus position may lead to femoral neck notching and damage to the retinacular vessels, impairing femoral head blood flow, which can be associated with early femoral neck fracture (Beaulé et al., 2006).*

Procedure

STEP 1

- A femoral head-neck elevator is used to facilitate preparation (Fig. 9).
- The femoral head is sized using a see-through gauge (Fig. 10). In the presence of osteophytes along the head-neck junction or in case of lack of anterior offset, the normal femoral neck axis needs to be re-established for proper drill guide pin placement using a high-speed burr and/or osteotomes (Fig. 11A and 11B). Careful attention must be paid to the retinacular vessels along the superior aspect of the neck (Fig. 12).
- Using the final-size cylindrical reamer (Fig. 13) or a pin-centering guide, the cylindrical reamer drill guide pin is then placed onto the femoral head with a 5–10° valgus orientation from the anatomic neck of the femur to give an angle between 135° and 145°.

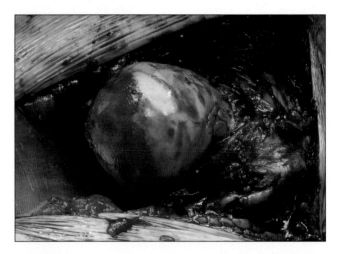

FIGURE 9

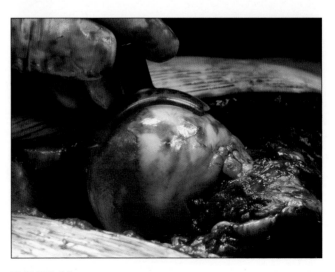

FIGURE 10

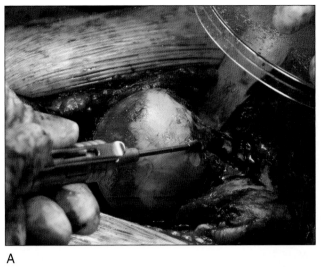

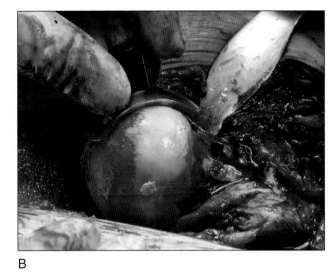

A

B

FIGURE 11

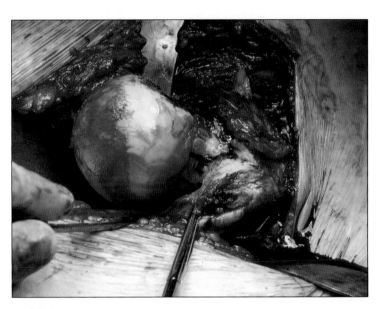

FIGURE 12

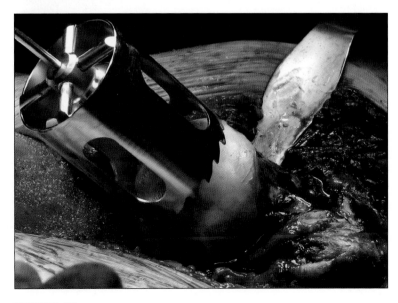

FIGURE 13

Instrumentation/ Implantation

• Femoral head-neck elevator

Controversies

• How close one should be to the femoral neck in terms of getting the smallest femoral component in order to preserve acetabular bone stock is uncertain.

■ In the sagittal plane, the guide pin is placed slightly superior and anterior to re-establish anterior head-neck offset and avoid reaming through the retinacular vessels.

■ The position of the guide pin is then checked for angulation with a goniometer with the leg in neutral rotation (Fig. 14). The appropriate cylindrical reamer gauge for the measured femoral head size should also be able to rotate freely around the guide to assure that the cylindrical reamer will not cause any neck notching (Fig. 15). The guide pin is repositioned as needed.

■ Cylindrical reaming is started with an oversized reamer that is two sizes bigger than the measured head. The reamer is advanced in longitudinal pulsatile fashion along the axis of the pin to avoid bending it.

■ Reaming is stopped 2–3 cm from the neck and a ¾-inch curved osteotome is used to remove any osteophytes (Fig. 16). The high-speed burr can be used to complete the preparation of the femoral head-neck junction, carefully avoid the retinacular vessels (Fig. 17).

■ Prior to proceeding, the direction of the cylindrical reamer compared to the anatomical neck should be re-evaluated and the guide pin adjusted as necessary.

■ The cylindrical reaming is then completed with the smaller reamers.

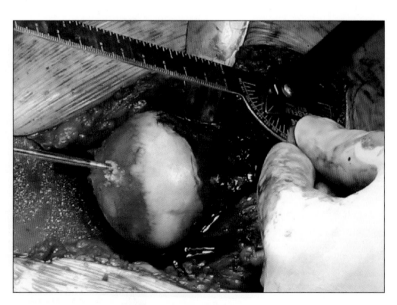

FIGURE 14

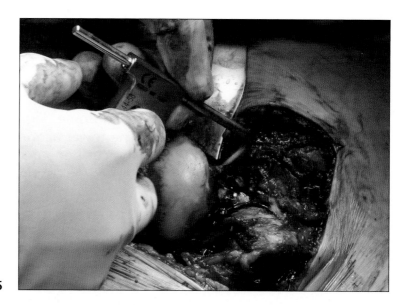

FIGURE 15

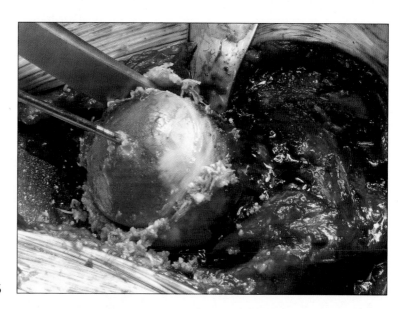

FIGURE 16

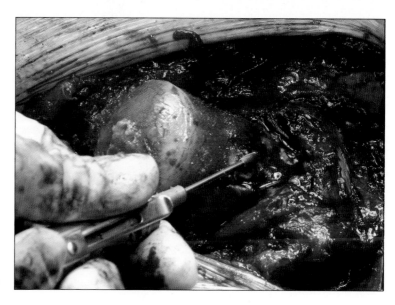

FIGURE 17

- A saw cutoff guide is placed over the reamed bone and is secured with two short pins through the guide holes, making sure that all of the reamed bone is covered.
- An oscillating saw is then used to resect the femoral head dome (Fig. 18).
- The tower alignment guide is then placed flush onto the cut bone and a final check of the orientation is carried out using a goniometer (Fig. 19).
- The stem hole is drilled (over-reaming by 2 mm is necessary for cemented stems to provide a cement mantle).
- The chamfer guide is subsequently placed into the drilled hole and the chamfer reamer is used to complete the femoral head preparation (Fig. 20).
- A trial prosthesis is used to confirm full seating (Fig. 21). It should rotate freely; any areas of asymmetric reaming are addressed with the final-size cylindrical reamer using the chamfer guide.
- Any cystic areas are removed using a curette.

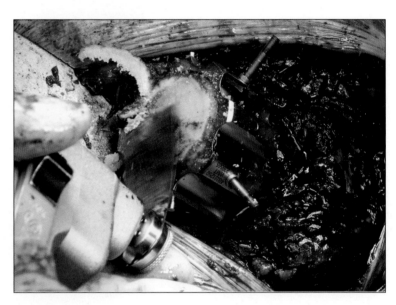

FIGURE 18

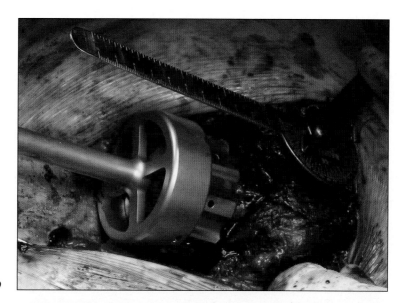

FIGURE 19

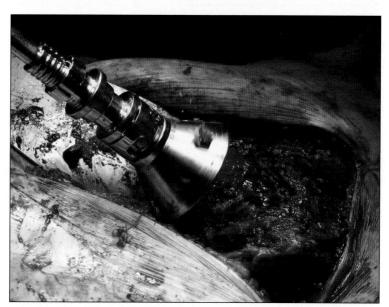

FIGURE 20

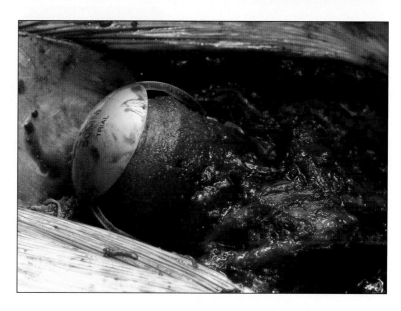

FIGURE 21

Instrumentation/ Implantation

• Padded Mayo stand
• Cobra retractor

Controversies

• If final acetabular preparation would entail going one size larger than one would usually do for a primary THR, is it better to downsize the femur or increase the socket size?

Step 2

■ With the femoral head preparation completed, the hip is placed in flexion and external rotation with the knee fully extended and resting onto a padded Mayo stand (Fig. 22).

■ A Cobra retractor is then placed onto the posterior wall of the acetabulum to retract the proximal femur, and a Hohmann retractor is placed on the anterior wall of the acetabulum to improve the exposure.

■ The anterior and posterior walls are assessed for any bony deficiency, and the labrum is excised with sharp dissection.

■ The inferomedial capsule is then released in a "pie crust" fashion using cautery to allow further mobilization of the femur.

■ The acetabulum is prepared in the usual fashion for a THR, starting with a reamer that is 8 mm smaller than the final size of the acetabular implant and ending with the last two reamers increasing in 1-mm increments. The Conserve Plus system has a 1-mm press-fit built into the component, allowing reaming up to the templated cup size.

■ Cysts are curettaged and grafted when encountered.

■ Acetabular preparation can be verified using a see-through gauge and metallic acetabular rings prior to implantation (Fig. 23).

■ The reamed acetabulum is then irrigated prior to inserting the component in 20° of anteversion and 45° of abduction. It is important to have the operative assistant help the surgeon in maintaining

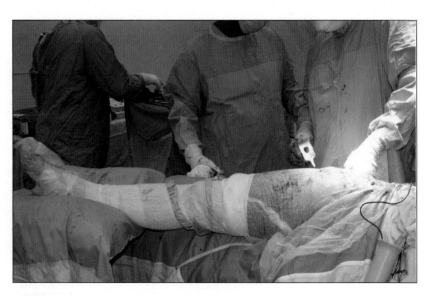

FIGURE 22

this alignment as the surgeon impacts the cup with a 10-lb hammer (Fig. 24). The cup is further impacted with the central ball impactor.

- The stability of the cup is then checked by pushing along its edges.
- Peripheral osteophytes are removed with an osteotome to prevent impingement.

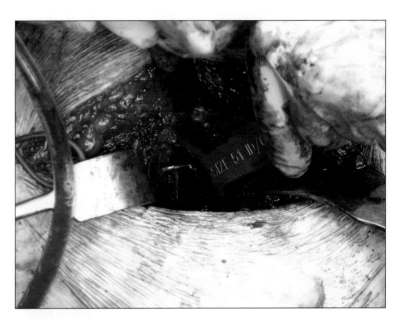

FIGURE 23

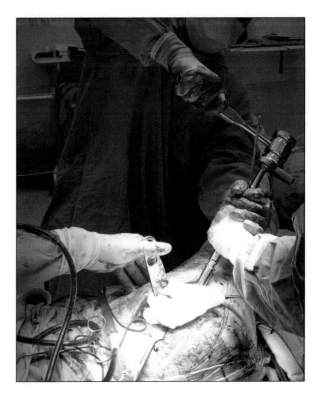

FIGURE 24

PEARLS

- *We recommend cementing the stem in patients with cystic defects greater than 1 cm or with a small femoral head (<46 mm) in order to increase the fixation area.*

- *Cover the femoral component with wet gauze as the cement is curing to prevent a large increase in temperature associated with thermal osteonecrosis.*

- *Avoid overfilling of the femoral component with cement.*

PITFALLS

- *Completely cleaning and drying the prepared femoral head prior to cementing is important in obtaining a good bone-cement interface and therefore solid fixation.*

- *Delaying implantation of the femoral component after cement mixing may compromise full seating of the component due to the high viscosity of the cement.*

Controversies

- Cementation of the short femoral stem
- Grafting or not grafting femoral head cysts

STEP 3

- With the hip in flexion and external rotation into a sterile cover, the femoral head is irrigated with pulsed lavage and dried using a tapered suction tip placed in the central drill guide hole (Fig. 25).
- Any area of hard cortical bone is cancellized using a ⅛-inch drill bit.
- The cement is poured in its liquid form to fill one quarter of the femoral component (Fig. 26).
- The prepared femoral head is further covered with cement without allowing cement to penetrate into the central drill guide hole, which is continuously being suctioned (Fig. 27).
- The femoral component is then cemented with continuous manual pressure as well as light impaction with a hammer (Fig. 28).
- Any excess cement is carefully removed using curettes (Fig. 29).
- Pressure is applied until the cement is fully cured.

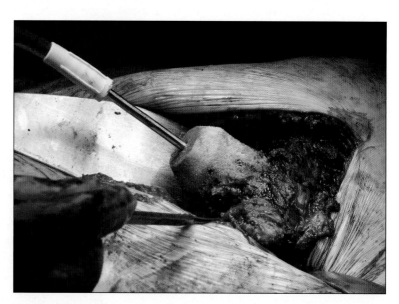

FIGURE 25

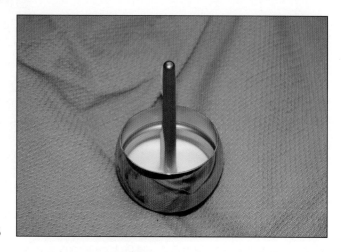

FIGURE 26

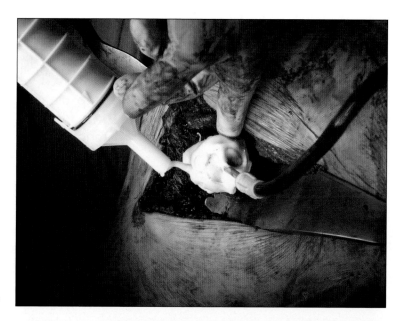

FIGURE 27

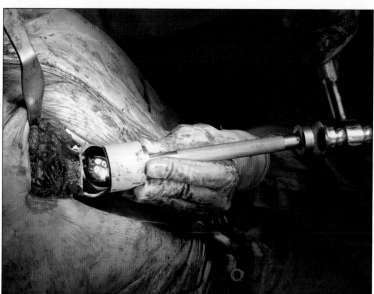

FIGURE 28

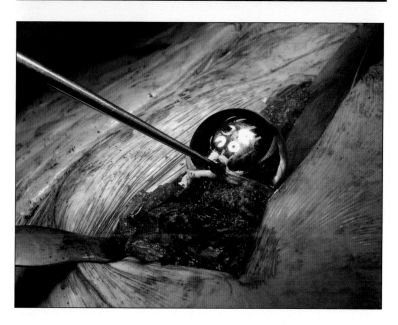

FIGURE 29

Step 4

- The hip is then reduced and taken through a ROM check to look for any bony impingement, which can be addressed with an osteotome.
- The capsule is closed using #1 interrupted Vicryl sutures and reattached to the acetabular rim posteriorly. Avoid watertight closure, which may lead to a hematoma buildup that can constrict the retinacular vessels at the head-neck junction.
- The GT osteotomy is subsequently properly reduced by placing a drill bit in the osteotomy site predrilled at the beginning of the procedure (Fig. 30). The reduction is further maintained with a large, sharp reduction forceps while a second hole is drilled and a 4.5-mm screw is placed to secure the reduction. A second screw is inserted for additional fixation. In cases of bilateral hip surgery, three screws are inserted in each hip.
- An intraoperative radiograph is taken to ensure proper screw and implant placement (Fig. 31).
- The incision is then closed in layered fashion without the use of drains.

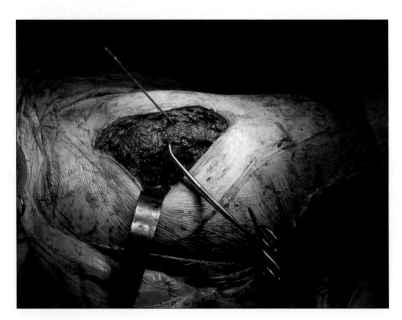

FIGURE 30

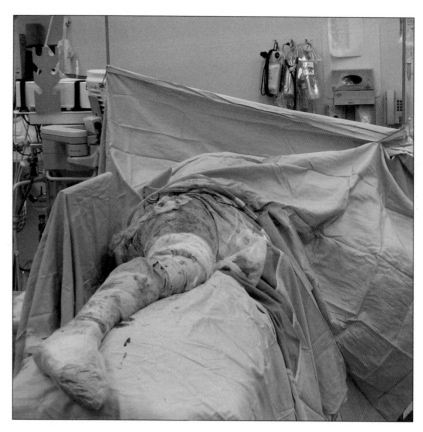

FIGURE 31

Controversies

• How active can patients be after hip resurfacing?

Postoperative Care and Expected Outcomes

- All patients are given antibiotic prophylaxis for 24 hours postoperatively as well as low-molecular-weight heparin for a period of 14 days.
- Patients are restricted to weight bearing of no more than 30 lbs with no active straight leg raise for 6 weeks.
- Patients are assessed by the hospital's physical therapist postoperatively and are given gait training and gentle ROM exercises to perform following discharge. At their first postoperative visit (6 weeks), the patients are started on formal physical therapy consisting of muscle-strengthening exercises.
- They are allowed to return to sports at the 3-month mark.

Evidence

Beaulé PE, Campbell PA, Hoke R, Dorey F. Notching of the femoral neck during resurfacing arthroplasty of the hip: a vascular study. J Bone Joint Surg Br. 2006;88:35–9.

Using laser Doppler flowmetry, femoral head blood flow was measured in 14 osteoarthritic femoral heads during routine total hip replacement surgery, before and after notching of the femoral neck. In ten hips there was a reduction in blood flow of more than 50% from the baseline value after simulated notching of the femoral neck. These results suggest that femoral head vascularity in the osteoarthritic state is similar to the non-arthritic state, where damage to the extraosseous vessels can predispose to avascular necrosis. Surgeons who perform resurfacing arthroplasty of the hip should pay careful attention to these vessels by avoiding excessive dissection around the femoral neck and/or notching. (Level I evidence)

Beaulé PE, Dorey FJ, LeDuff M, Gruen T, Amstutz HC. Risk factors affecting outcome of metal-on-metal surface arthroplasty of the hip. Clin Orthop Relat Res. 2004;(418):87–93.

Ninety-four hips in 83 patients with a mean age of 34.2 years (range, 15–40 years) were reviewed after undergoing metal-on-metal hip resurfacing. Seventy-one percent of the patients were males and 29% of the patients were females; 14% had previous surgery. The Chandler index and surface arthroplasty risk index were calculated. The mean follow-up at 3 years (range, 2–5 years) showed that three hips were converted to a total hip replacement at a mean of 27 months (range, 2–50 months) after the original surgery, and 10 hips had significant radiologic changes. The mean surface arthroplasty risk index for these 13 problematic hips versus the remaining hips was significantly higher, 4.7 and 2.6, respectively. With a surface arthroplasty risk index score greater than 3, the relative risk of early problems is 12 times greater than if surface arthroplasty risk index is less than or equal to 3. (Level III evidence)

Beaulé PE, Harvey N, Zaragoza E, Le Duff MJ, Dorey FJ. The femoral head/neck offset and hip resurfacing. J Bone Joint Surg Br. 2007;89B:9–15.

The femoral head/neck offset was measured in 63 hips undergoing metal-on-metal hip resurfacing and in 56 hips presenting with non-arthritic pain secondary to femoroacetabular impingement. Most hips undergoing resurfacing (57%; 36) had an offset ratio ≤0.15 preoperatively and required greater correction of offset at operation than the rest of the group. In the nonarthritic hips the mean offset ratio was 0.137 (0.04 to 0.23), with the offset ratio correlating negatively to an increasing alpha angle. An offset ratio ≤0.15 had a 9.5-fold increased relative risk of having an alpha angle ≥50.5°. Most hips undergoing resurfacing have an abnormal femoral head/neck offset, which is best assessed in the sagittal plane. (Level IV evidence)

Beaulé PE, Lee JL, Le Duff MJ, Amstutz HC, Ebramzadeh E. Orientation of the femoral component in surface arthroplasty of the hip. A biomechanical and clinical analysis. J Bone Joint Surg 2004;86A:2015–21.

The correlation between the orientation of the femoral component and the outcome of metal-on-metal hip resurfacing was evaluated, as were stresses within the resurfaced femoral head as a function of the orientation of the femoral component. Hips with a stem shaft angle of <130° had an increase in the relative risk of an adverse outcome by a factor of 6.1 (p < 0.004). In the entire cohort, stresses in the superior aspect of the resurfaced femoral head were substantially lower during slow walking than they were during fast walking (7.1 N/mm² compared with 14.2 N/mm²). Optimizing the femoral stem-shaft angle toward a valgus orientation during the preparation of the femoral head is important when a hip is being reconstructed with a surface arthroplasty because the resurfaced hip transmits the load through a narrow critical zone in the femoral head-neck region and the valgus angulation may reduce these stresses. (Level IV evidence)

Ganz R, Gill TJ, Gautier E, Ganz K, Krugel N, Berlemann U. Surgical dislocation of the adult hip a technique with full access to the femoral head and acetabulum without the risk of avascular necrosis. J Bone Joint Surg Br. 2001;83:1119–24.

A technique for operative dislocation of the hip, based on detailed anatomical studies of the blood supply is described. This surgical technique combines aspects of approaches which have been reported previously and consists of an anterior dislocation through a posterior approach with a "trochanteric flip" osteotomy. The external rotator muscles are not divided and the medial femoral circumflex artery is protected by the intact obturator externus. Initial experience using this approach in 213 hips over a period of seven years is reported with no cases of osteonecrosis. There is little morbidity associated with the technique and it allows the treatment of a variety of conditions, which may not respond well to other methods including arthroscopy. (Level IV evidence)

Gautier E, Ganz K, Krugel N, Gill T, Ganz R. Anatomy of the medial femoral circumflex artery and its surgical implications. J Bone Joint Surg Br. 2000;82:679–83.

The anatomy of the MFCA and its branches were described based on dissections of 24 cadaver hips after injection of neoprene-latex into the femoral or internal iliac arteries. They demonstrated that obturator externus protects the deep branch of the MFCA from being disrupted or stretched during dislocation of the hip in any direction after serial release of all other soft-tissue attachments of the proximal femur, including a complete circumferential capsulotomy. Precise knowledge of the extracapsular anatomy of the MFCA and its surrounding structures will help to avoid iatrogenic avascular necrosis of the head of the femur in reconstructive surgery of the hip. (Level IV evidence)

REVISION TOTAL HIP ARTHROPLASTY

SECTION III

Digital Templating for Revision Total Hip Arthroplasty

Mahmoud A. Hafez and Emil H. Schemitsch

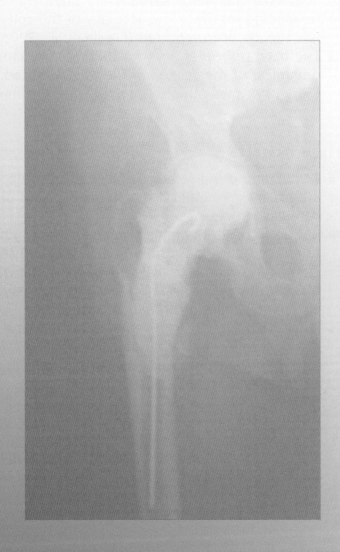

Introduction

- Procedure 4, on templating for primary total hip arthroplasty (THA), outlined the basics of templating and the specific technical steps for primary procedures. This chapter is focused on the specific technical details for templating in revision THA and provides some practical examples.
- At St. Michael's Hospital in Toronto, we routinely use the EndoMap software system (Siemens AG, Medical Solutions, Erlangen, Germany) for preoperative templating for THA. The accuracy of this software has already been reported (Davila et al., 2006).
- The basic principles of templating are the same regardless of the version of the software used, and these principles can also be applied to traditional templating.

Indications

- Templating is indicated for every revision hip arthroplasty, whether it is a straightforward or a complicated case.
- Revision THA is a complex procedure with a higher risk of complications and unforeseen circumstances. Templating is an essential part of preoperative planning that is more important and sophisticated for revision than for primary arthroplasty.
- Preoperative planning is required for the type of implants to be used, the method of fixation (cemented, uncemented, or hybrid), and the need for bone grafting and/or special instruments or devices.
  - Larger femoral heads or constrained cups may be required if a higher risk of dislocation is expected.
  - In revision surgery, bone stock is usually deficient, and metal or allograft augmentation may be required. It is useful to know in advance the cup size and the level of femoral neck cut to facilitate minimal bone removal.
  - The anatomy is usually distorted in revision surgery, and planning is required to restore the center of rotation, offset, and leg length and to obtain optimal alignment of the implants.
- Templating may allow the surgeon to predict intraoperative difficulties and possible complications.

- Implant inventory is another concern. Revision implants and instrumentation are not usually stored at the hospital site. Surgeons, nurses, and manufacturers need to be aware long in advance about unusual implants or instruments.
- The value of preoperative planning for revision THA has been reported by several authors (Barrack and Burnett, 2006; Bono, 2004; Knight and Atwater, 1992; Morrey, 1992; Seel et al., 2006).

Examination/Imaging

- History, clinical examination and laboratory investigations are essential components of preoperative planning and should be done routinely before templating.
  - Information about previous THA (ipsilateral and/or contralateral) should be obtained from old hospital notes.
  - Measurements for leg length discrepancy should be done clinically and radiologically. Patients should be asked if they are aware of leg length discrepancy. Measure leg lengths and account for pelvic obliquity and flexion deformity.
- Good-quality radiographs are essential and should include anteroposterior and lateral views extending beyond the tip of the femoral component and the cement restrictor. The position of the patient and the leg during radiographic examination is critical (see Pitfalls).
- Templating for revision procedures should be done in the outpatient clinic and should be repeated just before surgery to take into consideration any changes that may have occurred during the waiting time for surgery.

Positioning/Exposures

- The technical steps for templating are the same whether a posterior or a lateral approach is used and whether the patient is positioned on his or her side or supine.

Procedure

- If templating is found to be practically difficult on the affected side, the opposite normal hip can be used for templating. The determined center of rotation on the affected side can be transferred to the normal side.

STEP 1: RADIOGRAPHIC ASSESSMENT

- Look at bone quality, evidence of loosening, osteolysis, cortical thinning, perforation, fractures, implant migration or failure. Look at the polyethylene liner and find out if there is any evidence for polyethylene wear The radiographic assessment of a failed THA in Figure 1 shows loosening of the acetabular component with polyethylene wear and osteolysis of the proximal femur.
- For two-stage revision procedures, it may be useful to do a preliminary templating before the removal of the failed component and then a final templating before the second stage of the procedure. Figure 2 shows a preoperative radiograph before a second-stage revision, with the cement spacer in place and the deficient medial femoral cortex that requires a femoral stem with calcar replacement.
- Make a preliminary decision on what type of implants are to be used, whether cemented, cementless, or hybrid implants.
- Decide whether distal or proximal loading stems are to be used.
- If a decision is made to revise one component, the surgeon needs to find a suitable new implant compatible with the retained component.
- Information about the manufacturer and the sizes of the old implants can be found in the hospital notes, particularly in the stick-on labels from the manufacturers.

STEP 2: CORRECT RADIOGRAPHIC MAGNIFICATION

- Eliminate magnification by scaling the anteroposterior (AP) pelvic radiograph using the software facilities.
- Consult radiographers about the percentage of magnification, and be aware that the degree of magnification is related to patient size. Conn et al. (2002) described a simple technique using a coin to determine radiographic magnification.

PITFALLS

- *Radiographic magnification is variable and depends on the radiographic techniques used and the patient's size.*

- *Errors in correcting magnification will result in wrong selection of implant types and sizes.*

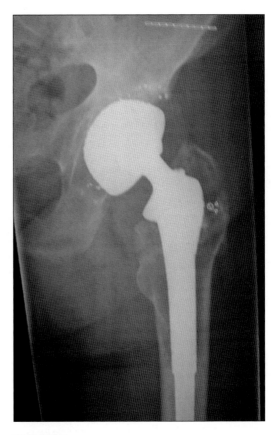

FIGURE 1

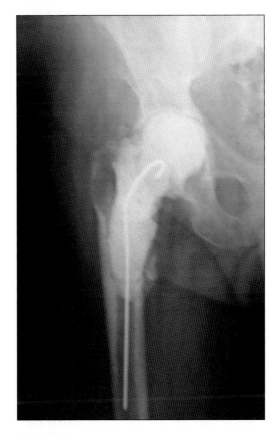

FIGURE 2

■ In case of traditional templating, the printed acetates are usually magnified and the percentage of magnification is usually printed on the acetates.

STEP 3: MEASURE LEG LENGTH DISCREPANCY

■ Measure leg length discrepancy using fixed landmarks such as the lesser trochanters, greater trochanters, or teardrops.
■ The software of a digital templating system can automatically calculate the leg length discrepancy.
■ Compare between radiographic and clinical measurements and differentiate between true and apparent discrepancy.
■ Repeat clinical and radiographic measurements and record the final discrepancy in millimeters.

STEP 4: TEMPLATE THE ACETABULAR COMPONENT

■ Use the long unilateral AP radiograph to template for THA implants.
■ Identify landmarks such as the ilioischial line, teardrop, acetabular margins, center of rotation, and greater and lesser trochanter.
■ Start with acetabular templating.
■ First select the desired cup from the implant library and then modify the size and position to fit the acetabulum. A larger cup is usually selected to compensate for bone loss. The sizing of the cup may help in restoring the center of rotation by avoiding the use of a smaller implant that may lead to a high hip center.
■ Place the cup in a near-anatomic position to reproduce the center of rotation. If the cup is placed proximal or distal to this, then shortening or lengthening of the leg will be seen. Align the cup according to the required angle for abduction (e.g., 45°). Consider minimal bone removal and sufficient bone coverage laterally. Use the ilioischial line and the teardrop as landmarks and position the cup lateral to the teardrop.
■ For a cemented cup, allow enough space for an adequate cement mantle. Estimate the volume of the cavity in the superolateral part of the false acetabulum. This volume should be reproduced intraoperatively, and the defect must be filled by the appropriate material (bone graft, cement, or metal).
■ Figure 3 shows the templating for both acetabular and femoral components with the correction of shortening resulting from the dislocation of the cement spacer.

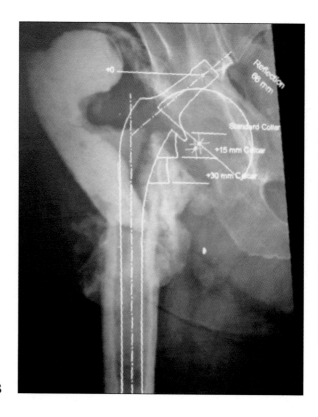

FIGURE 3

Step 5: Template the Femoral Component

- Select the desired stem from the implant library.
  Modify the size and position to fit the femoral canal.
  Figure 4 shows templating of the femoral component
  in the presence of a fractured femoral stem.

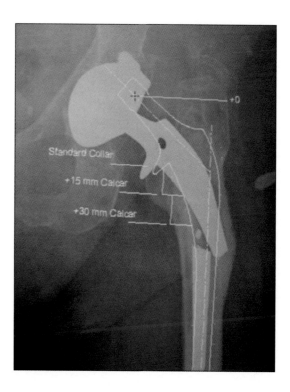

FIGURE 4

- Compare different offsets (standard or high) to find a better match for the patient's original offset.
- A calcar replacement may be required, and the height of the calcar can be determined by measuring the distance between the stem collar and the available calcar. Allograft may be considered if bone loss is excessive (>30 mm).
- Determine the proper offset.
- Try to use a femoral stem with a zero head to leave you with the flexibility to increase or decrease length intraoperatively and obtain optimal soft tissue tension.
- The stem length should bypass cortical defects.
- Lateral radiographs may provide useful information with respect to the position of the existing femoral stem, the quality of bone, and the degree of femoral anteversion and whether there is excessive ante- or retroversion. They also help in localizing areas of loosening, osteolysis, cortical thinning, perforation, fractures, or implant failure. The images also show the shape of the femoral canal and the degree of bowing as well as the entry point and expected alignment of the stem.

STEP 6: CORRECT LEG LENGTH DISCREPANCY AND MEASURE THE LENGTH OF NECK RESECTION

- Adjust the height of the femoral stem to correct leg length discrepancy based on the center of rotation of the acetabulum.
  - In case there is no preoperative leg length discrepancy, the center of the head should be at the same level as that of the acetabulum.
  - In case of preoperative shortening, the center of the head should be elevated above the center of the cup by the amount of required lengthening in millimeters. For example, if the shortening was 20 mm, the center of the head should be placed vertically 20 mm above the center of the cup.
- It may be difficult to obtain full correction of leg length discrepancy, Barrack and Burnett (2006) recommend correcting only two thirds of shortening, since it is difficult to overcome excessive soft tissue tension associated with chronic shortening.
- Measure the femoral neck cut, the distance between the lesser trochanter and stem collar (or to the medial border of a collarless stem).
- Measure the length of the femoral neck resection in relation to the lesser trochanter using a digital ruler. This measurement should be reproduced intraoperatively.

- Measure the position of the shoulder tip of the prosthesis in relation to the tip of the greater trochanter using a digital ruler. This measurement should be checked intraoperatively.
- Measure the center of the femoral head in relation to the greater trochanter. This measurement should be checked intraoperatively.

Outcome Data and Operative Application

- The computer screen displays the relevant information regarding the implants, such as component sizes, stem length, offset, neck height, neck length, and the like. In Figure 5, the computer screen shows the templating of a distal-loading femoral component and complete data from the manufacturer on the selected implant.
- The entire plan can be saved as an electronic file or printed and attached to the patient notes, thus providing a permanent record for clinical, research, audit, or inventory (reordering) purposes.
- Inform nursing staff about sizes of templated implants and any change in plan or type of implants.
- The relevant information should be recorded by the surgeon and used during surgery.

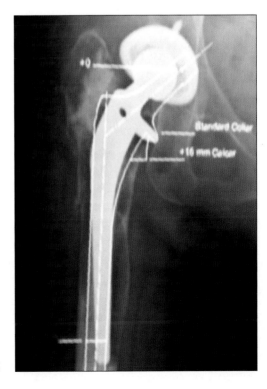

FIGURE 5

- During surgery, the surgeon should adequately expose the lesser trochanter and mark the level of neck resection according to the preoperative templating.
- Prepare the acetabulum and the femur for the types and sizes of the implants predetermined by templating.
- It is not unusual to deviate from the plan and select sizes above or below the predetermined sizes.
- The soft tissue tension and the stability of the joint are another variable that should be borne in mind. Stability should not be compromised at the expense of leg length equality; further adjustment of the level of the femoral stem with the selection of the appropriate femoral neck length (head) may be required to optimize the stability of the hip joint.

Evidence

Barrack RL, Burnett RS. Preoperative planning for revision total hip arthroplasty. Instr Course Lect. 2006;55:233–44.

In an instructional course lecture, the authors emphasized that preoperative planning for revision THA can anticipate potential complications, help to reduce surgical time, minimize risks, decrease the stress level of the entire surgical team, and increase the rate of successful outcomes for patients.

Bono JV. Digital templating in total hip arthroplasty. J Bone Joint Surg [Am]. 2004;86(Suppl 2):118–22.

In a review article, the use of digital planning for THA was recommended, as it was found fast, precise, and cost-efficient. Also, it provided a permanent record of the templating process.

Conn KS, Clarke MT, Hallett JP. A simple guide to determine the magnification of radiographs and to improve the accuracy of preoperative templating. J Bone Joint Surg [Br]. 2002;84:269–72.

The authors reported radiographic magnification may vary despite using standardized radiological techniques, thus giving misleading measurements during templating. A coin was used to calculate the magnification, with significant improvement in the accuracy of templating (p = 0.05).

Davila JA, Kransdorf MJ, Duffy GP. Surgical planning of total hip arthroplasty: accuracy of computer-assisted EndoMap software in predicting component size. Skeletal Radiol. 2006;35:390–3.

The authors reviewed the results of EndoMap Software in templating primary THA and found 72% of femoral component sizing was within one size of that used, and 94% within two sizes. The acetabular component sizing was more accurate with 86% within one component size and 94% within two component sizes.

Knight JL, Atwater RD. Preoperative planning for total hip arthroplasty: quantitating its utility and precision. J Arthroplasty. 1992;7(Suppl):403–9.

Surgeons recorded the preoperative plan and the surgical events of 110 consecutive primary THA, and found a need to introduce better methods to estimate magnification and bone morphology from preoperative radiographs.

Morrey BF: Instability after total hip arthroplasty. Orthop Clin North Am. 1992;23:237–48.

The author reported a dislocation rate as high as 25% after revision THR surgery. The most reliable surgical procedure for dislocation was reorientation of the retroverted acetabular component. The author advised to define the precise cause of the instability and plan the surgery accordingly.

Seel MJ, Hafez MA, Eckman K, Jaramaz B, Davidson D, DiGioia AM. 3-D planning and virtual x-ray in revision hip arthroplasty for instability. Clin Orthop Relat Res. 2006;(442):35–8.

The authors used sophisticated computer assisted techniques (such as navigation systems) for 3-D preoperative planning in a revision total hip arthroplasty for recurrent dislocation. Problems such as impingement, cup malpositioning, bone deficiency and integrity of fixation screws were assessed. The system allowed accurate planning and optimal orientation of the acetabular implant.

REVISION TOTAL HIP ARTHROPLASTY: EXPOSURES

Extended Trochanteric Osteotomy: Posterior Approach

Scott M. Sporer and Wayne G. Paprosky

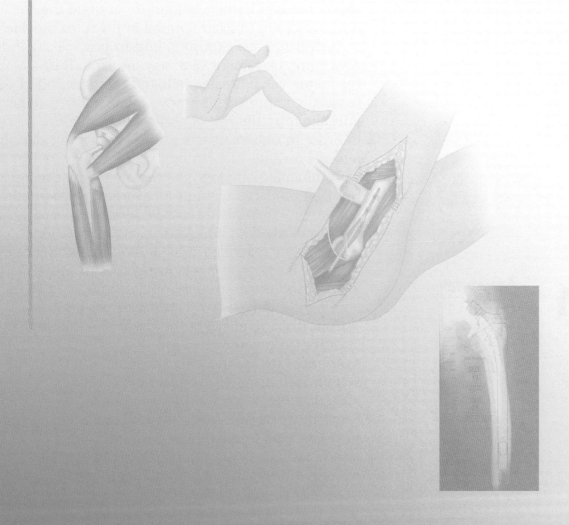

Introduction

- Total hip arthroplasty can provide predictable pain relief and improve function in patients with degenerative arthritis, and is now recognized as one of the most cost-effective surgical interventions. Despite the overwhelming success and long-term reliability of total hip arthroplasty, several situations necessitate the revision of the femoral component.
- The use of an extended trochanteric osteotomy allows exposure of the proximal femur through the use of a controlled cortical fracture. This surgical technique is extremely helpful to facilitate the removal of a well-fixed femoral implant, to provide increased surgical exposure, and to provide concentric placement of a new implant. This technique will ultimately minimize undersizing of the femoral components, improve initial implant stability, and minimize the risk of cortical perforation.
- In order to obtain a successful surgical result during femoral revision, the femoral stem must be removed with minimal bone loss, the remaining host bone must be prepared without inadvertent perforation, and a femoral implant must be inserted concentrically with adequate axial and rotational stability. The extended trochanteric osteotomy can facilitate these goals by allowing
  - Improved access to the implant-bone or implant-cement interface
  - Concentric reaming of the distal femur in patients with proximal femoral deformity
  - Appropriate abductor tensioning
  - Improved acetabular visualization
  - Predictable healing of the osteotomy
- Familiarity with this surgical technique is crucial for surgeons who frequently perform revision arthroplasty or primary total hip arthroplasty in patients with proximal femoral deformity.

Indications

- In general, an extended trochanteric osteotomy should be performed if it is contemplated by the surgeon.
- Common indications:
  - A well-fixed implant may require removal because of sepsis, recurrent dislocation due to femoral component malposition and/or inadequate offset,

a poor track record, or the need to improve acetabular exposure. Removal of a well-fixed femoral implant can be very challenging. Extensive bone loss can occur while attempting to remove a well-fixed implant due to the inability to disrupt the bone-prosthesis interface distally with proximal exposure alone. While a cortical window can be helpful, this technique will weaken the remaining host bone and require a longer stem to bypass the stress riser.

- The removal of retained distal cement may be necessary, and is equally challenging. Isolated proximal exposure has been shown to result in a higher prevalence of cortical perforation while attempting to remove distal cement. The length of the extended trochanteric osteotomy can be planned to allow easy visual access to the distal cement plug such that standard drills, taps, and curettes can be used to disrupt the bone-cement interface and facilitate the removal of retained cement.

- Proximal femoral varus remodeling is observed in up to 30% of patients with a loose femoral stem. While component extraction may be relatively easy in these patients, the subsequent surgical reconstruction is challenging due to the deformed proximal bone.

  ◆ The surgical options in patients with proximal femoral deformity include accepting the deformity and cementing a femoral component into the deformity or performing an extended trochanteric osteotomy, which will allow concentric reaming of the femoral canal.

  ◆ Cementing a femoral stem into a varus-remodeled femur is recommended only in a low-demand patient due to the poor results of cement femoral revisions. Attempting to insert an extensively coated stem in a patient with varus remodeling without the use of an extended trochanteric osteotomy will result in a high prevalence of cortical perforation, undersizing of the femoral component, and a varus malposition.

■ Additional relative indications:

- Need for improved acetabular exposure either due to heterotopic bone formation or in severe acetabular deficiencies requiring extensive visualization of the anterior and posterior column

- Use during femoral revision in patients with severe trochanteric osteolysis to minimize inadvertent fracture
- Rarely, use in the primary setting in patients with prior osteotomies, malunions, or proximal femoral deformity due to congenital dysplasias

Examination/Imaging

■ Standard anteroposterior (AP) radiographs of the pelvis and AP and lateral radiographs of the femur are required for preoperative planning of and extended trochanteric osteotomy. The AP pelvis radiograph can be used to estimate the leg length discrepancy, while the AP radiograph of the femur can be used to determine the apex of the deformity in a varus-remodeled femur and plan the appropriate length of the osteotomy.

Surgical Anatomy

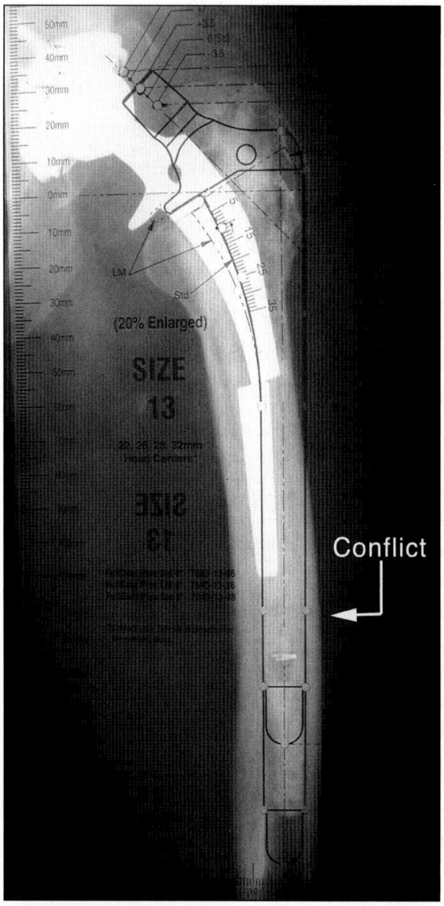

■ The length of the osteotomy will be dependent upon the indication.
  - Varus remodeling of the proximal femur will occur in up to 30% of femoral revisions and is most frequently observed at the tip of a loose femoral stem. Due to the remodeling, neutral component alignment cannot be achieved from a proximal starting position. The inability to place a femoral component in neutral position due to varus remodeling has been termed a *conflict* (Fig. 1). In these situations, the length of the extended trochanteric osteotomy should extend at least to the apex of the deformity. Failure to reach the level of the deformity will necessitate that the femoral preparation remain in a varus alignment.
  - When the extended trochanteric osteotomy is performed for removal of retained distal cement, the length will need to be within a few centimeters of the distal cement plug. A shorter osteotomy can be performed if the indication is to improve surgical exposure or if a loose distal cement mantle is present. However, a sufficient length of cortical bone below the lesser trochanter is required in order to securely reattach the osteotomy fragment at the completion of the procedure. A minimum of two cables is required to securely fix the trochanteric fragment at the completion of the procedure.

FIGURE 1

- The length of the osteotomy is also dependent upon the implant chosen for the reconstruction.
  - Preoperative templates are essential in deciding the length of the osteotomy in order to obtain a stable implant. If an extensively porous coated stem is used, a minimum of 4–5 cm of "scratch fit" will be required in order to obtain sufficient axial and rotational stability. If a tapered stem is chosen, it is important that the osteotomy does not extend past the distal metaphyseal/diaphyseal flare.
  - Once the position of the osteotomy is marked, the location of the transverse limb is measured from a fixed bony landmark such as the tip of the greater trochanter (Fig. 2A and 2B) or the lesser trochanter.

PEARLS

- *The length of the extended trochanteric osteotomy should be minimized to use the shortest femoral revision stem possible yet should be long enough to bypass the apex of the femoral remodeling, to achieve component/cement removal, and to allow at least two cerclage cables to be placed around the osteotomy.*

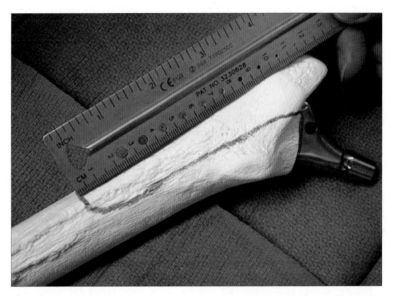

A

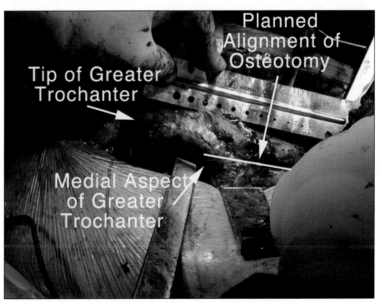

FIGURE 2 B

Instrumentation

- An oscillating saw with a narrow blade is required for the longitudinal limb, while a "pencil-tip" burr is required for the transverse limb of the osteotomy.
- Several wide osteotomes are required to distribute stress along the trochanteric fragment while the osteotomy is being completed.
- Depending upon the indication for the osteotomy, a metal cutting burr may be required to section a well-fixed extensively porous coated stem before a Gigli saw can be used to remove the proximal portion of the stem and cylindrical trephines be used to remove the distal portion of the stem.
- Reverse hooks, cement drills, and osteotomes will be required to remove well-fixed distal cement.
- A minimum of two cerclage wires/cables are required to securely fix the osteotomy fragment upon completion of the procedure.

Positioning

- When performing the osteotomy, the hip is placed in extension and internal rotation with the knee flexed. This position will minimize the risk of a traction injury to the sciatic nerve yet allow exposure of the posterior aspect of the femur.

Portals/Exposures

- The surgical approach in the revision setting may be directed by previous surgical incisions. We prefer to use a posterolateral approach, which allows both proximal and distal extension and provides excellent visualization of both the femur and the acetabulum.
- The patient is placed in a lateral decubitus position, taking care to stabilize the pelvis with positioners along the sacrum and pubic symphysis.
- A lateral surgical skin incision is made in line with the femur over the posterior third of the greater trochanter. The tensor fascia lata and the fascia of the gluteus maximus are then split in line with the surgical incision and retracted with a Charnley retractor.
- The posterior border of the gluteus maximus tendon is identified and retracted anteriorly. The posterior pseudocapsule and the short external rotators are then elevated as a posteriorly based flap. Elevating these structures as a flap will allow a posterior capsular repair at the completion of the surgery.
- A portion of the gluteus maximus insertion is released to allow mobilization of the femur. The femoral head is now dislocated posteriorly when the hip is placed in flexion and internal rotation. The knee remains flexed to decrease tension on the sciatic nerve.
- The soft tissue surrounding the proximal portion of the femoral stem is removed and the stability of the femoral component is assessed. If the stem is grossly loose and the greater trochanter is not preventing extrication, the component is removed. However, if the trochanter is preventing component removal or if the stem is well fixed, an in situ extended trochanteric osteotomy should be performed.
- An in situ osteotomy should also be considered if hip dislocation is difficult due to severe acetabular protrusion or extensive heterotopic bone formation.

Procedure

STEP 1

- The posterior margin of the vastus lateralis is identified and the muscle belly is mobilized anteriorly off of the lateral femur while attempting to minimize soft tissue stripping.
- A Chandler or Hohmann retractor is placed around the femoral shaft at the desired length of the osteotomy, exposing the underlying periosteum. The insertion of the gluteus maximus tendon is preserved unless release is required to mobilize the femur for visualization.

STEP 2

- The position of the proposed osteotomy can now be marked with either electrocautery or a pen. The tip of the greater trochanter can be used as a landmark or, if the femoral stem has been removed, this can be used to determine the length of the osteotomy.
- A sagittal saw is directed from posterolateral to anterolateral beginning anterior to the linea aspera while the femur remains in full extension and internal rotation. Ideally, the osteotomy fragment should encompass the posterolateral third of the proximal femur and should be oriented perpendicular to the anteversion of the hip (Fig. 3A and 3B).
- If the femoral component has been previously extracted, the oscillating saw can then be guided toward the far anterolateral cortex, where the cortical bone can be "etched" to facilitate a greenstick-type fracture. If the femoral component is retained, the oscillating saw must be angled anterolaterally in an attempt to maximize the width of the osteotomy yet avoid hitting the retained femoral component.
- Proximally, the saw is angled posteromedially so that the entire greater trochanter is released with the osteotomy.

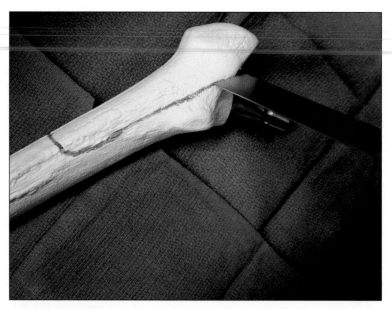

A

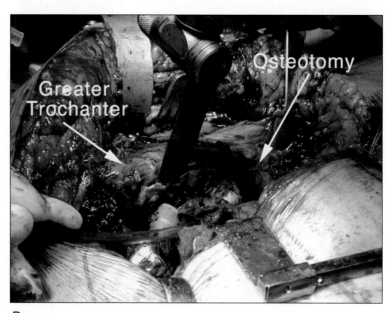

B

FIGURE 3

Step 3

- The distal transverse limb of the osteotomy should be made with the use of a pencil-tip burr (Fig. 4). The corners of the osteotomy should be rounded to eliminate a stress riser and decrease the risk of propagating a distal fracture.
- An oscillating saw or the pencil-tip burr can be used to initiate the distal anterior limb of the osteotomy.

Step 4

- Multiple wide Lambotte osteotomes are used to gently lever the osteotomy site from posterior to anterior (Fig. 5A and 5B).

Pearls

- *When levering the osteotomy anteriorly, multiple wide osteotomes should be used simultaneously to distribute the stress along the greatest distance.*

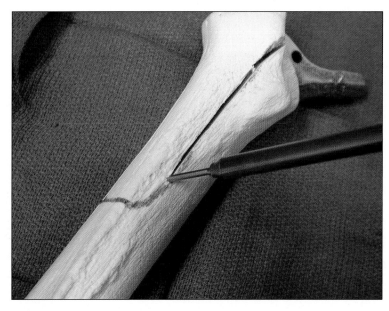

FIGURE 4

- The entire osteotomy fragment should be moved as a unit to avoid fracture at the level of the vastus ridge. Once the anterior limb of the osteotomy has been initiated, the trochanteric fragment can be retracted anteriorly with the attached abductors and vastus lateralis.
- The tight pseudocapsule along the anterior aspect of the greater trochanter must be released while mobilizing the osteotomy fragment in order to avoid inadvertent fracture of the greater trochanter.

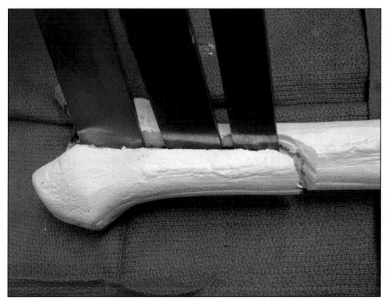

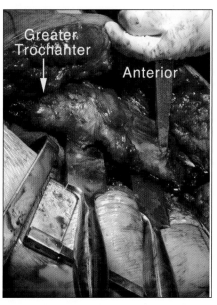

A

B

FIGURE 5

- Since the blood supply and innervation to the vastus enter anteriorly, it is important to minimize dissection along the anterolateral limb of the osteotomy.

STEP 5

- If the femoral component was extracted prior to the osteotomy, the pseudomembrane within the femur can now be removed.
- If cement had previously been used, a high-speed burr along with cement splitters can be used to remove the retained cement and the distal plug. Cement remaining on the trochanteric fragment is retained until the end of the procedure in order to strengthen the often compromised trochanteric bone during surgical retraction.
- If an osteotomy was required to remove a well-fixed proximally coated implant, a pencil-tip burr can now be utilized to expose the implant-bone interface around the majority of the implant. A Gigli saw can then be placed around the proximal femur and be used to disrupt the bone-prosthesis interface before the component removal.
- If the osteotomy was required to remove a well-fixed extensively coated stem, the stem can now be transected with a metal cutting burr at the junction between the tapered and cylindrical portion of the implant. The proximal portion of the implant can be removed as described above while the remaining distal cylindrical portion of the stem can be removed with the use of a trephine 0.5 mm larger than the implanted stem.

STEP 6: BONE PREPARATION

- Once the previous femoral component has been successfully removed, any remaining pseudomembrane or cement should be removed with the use of a reverse hook in order to minimize the risk of inadvertent femoral fracture during femoral preparation.
- A distal pedestal is often observed in loose cementless implants and should also be removed to allow concentric femoral reaming.
- The vast majority of femoral revisions are performed using a cementless implant that relies upon distal fixation. Depending upon the pattern of bone loss, the patient's anatomy, and the length of the osteotomy, either a bowed or a straight extensively coated stem or a distally tapered stem may be chosen.

- Flexible reamers are used to prepare the canal when a curved extensively coated stem is chosen, while a solid straight reamer is used when a straight extensively coated stem is chosen.
- The femoral canal is sequentially reamed until cortical resistance is encountered.
  - The femoral canal is under-reamed by 0.5 mm to allow axial and rotation stability once the slightly larger implant is inserted. Throughout the reaming, the surgeon should be aware of the depth and the approximate location of the new stem.
  - A minimum of 5 cm of diaphyseal bone, scratch fit, is required when utilizing a fully porous coated stem. Alternative methods of reconstruction, such as a tapered stem, should be considered if this amount of scratch fit is not feasible.
- Once significant endosteal resistance is encountered with the reamers, a femoral trial can be placed. The hip can then be reduced and brought through a range of motion to assess stability.
- Provided the hip is stable, the amount of required femoral anteversion is marked. If a curved 8-inch or 10-inch stem is utilized, the bow of the femur and the prosthesis will control the ultimate amount of femoral anteversion. If the bowed implant does not allow adequate anteversion and the hip is not stable in this configuration, alternative methods of reconstruction, such as a modular stem, should be considered.

PEARLS

• *A prophylactic cerclage can be placed distal to the osteotomy before femoral preparation and stem insertion to minimize the risk of fracture.*

STEP 7: PROSTHESIS IMPLANTATION

■ The placement of a fully porous coated stem in the revision situation is similar to that used during primary arthroplasty. Figure 6 shows a femoral reconstruction with an extensively coated femoral stem. Note the healing of the osteotomy and the neutral alignment of the femoral stem.

■ A hole gauge should be utilized to verify that the manufacturing process has resulted in the appropriate distal femoral diameter. (For example, an 18-mm component should be able to pass through the 18.25-mm hole and not the 18.00-mm hole.) If the component is slightly oversized, the femoral canal can be reamed an additional 0.5 mm to avoid femoral fracture.

■ A prophylactic cerclage wire can be placed distal to the osteotomy site in order to minimize hoop stresses during component insertion and minimize the risk of fracture propagation. Additionally, the introitis at the level of the osteotomy can be reamed line to line for a length of approximately 1 cm to minimize the risk of fracture.

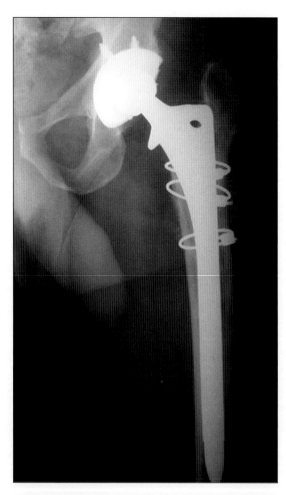

FIGURE 6

■ The femoral component should now be able to be inserted manually within 4–5 cm of the desired depth. If the implant must be seated more than 5 cm, the canal should be reamed line to line.

■ A series of gentle blows are used to seat the implant while in the appropriate amount of anteversion. Ideally, the stem should advance with each strike of the mallet and require 20–30 impacts until fully seated.

Step 8: Wound Closure

■ Any cement adherent to the trochanteric fragment should be removed once the femoral stem is fully seated.

■ The leg is placed in slight abduction and internal rotation during reattachment of the osteotomy fragment.

■ A minimum of two cables or wires is needed to secure the greater trochanteric fragment to the remaining femoral shaft.

■ A high-speed barrel burr may be required to shape the trochanteric fragment in order to allow the osteotomy to rest against the lateral shoulder of the prosthesis and maximize bony apposition to the femoral shaft. The trochanteric fragment will not be able to have bone apposition both anteriorly and posteriorly in situations in which the extended trochanteric osteotomy was performed due to varus femoral remodeling. In these situations, the osteotomy should be advanced slightly distally and posteriorly to improve stability and minimize impingement during internal rotation.

■ The cables around the osteotomy are tightened from distally to proximally with a decreasing amount of force. Care must be taken to avoid a trochanteric fracture at the level of the vastus ridge.

■ Bone grafting of the osteotomy site is not routinely performed unless host bone from the reamings of the acetabulum or femur is available.

■ Our preference is to repair the posterior capsule and short external rotators to the posterior aspect of the gluteus medius.

■ The gluteus maximus fascia and the iliotibial band are closed over a drain with a nonabsorbable #1 suture while the subcutaneous tissue is closed with an absorbable 2-0 suture.

PEARLS

• *The osteotomy fragment should be advanced distally and posteriorly before securing it to the remaining shaft of the femur. This will provide appropriate abductor tension and minimize the risk of impingement.*

Postoperative Care and Expected Outcomes

- Patients who have undergone a femoral revision may be treated with an abduction orthosis for 6–8 weeks postoperatively to minimize the risk of instability. During this time, they are 30% weight bearing on the operative leg utilizing a walker or crutch for ambulation.
- At the end of 6–8 weeks, they are converted to a cane and advance their weight bearing as tolerated.
- Patients are instructed to avoid active abduction for 6–12 weeks until radiographic evidence of healing at the osteotomy site is present.

CLINICAL RESULTS
- The senior author has previously reported his results when using an extended trochanteric osteotomy during revision femoral surgery.
  - From 1992 to 1996, 142 consecutive hip revisions were performed encompassing an extended trochanteric osteotomy; 122 patients were able to be followed at an average of 2.6 years.
  - There were no nonunions of the osteotomized fragments and no cases of proximal migration greater than 2 mm. Radiographically, all cases demonstrated bony union by 3 months.
  - This cohort of patients was re-evaluated with additional patients from 1992 to 1998. At an average 3.9-year follow-up, there were two nonunions (1.2%) and one malunion (0.6%). The remaining osteotomies achieved bony union.
- Other surgeons have seen similar clinical results with the use of an extended trochanteric osteotomy. Chen et al. reported a 98% union rate in 46 hips when an extended trochanteric osteotomy was used during revision surgery.

COMPLICATIONS
- Potential complications with the use of an extended trochanteric osteotomy include proximal migration, nonunion or malunion of the osteotomy fragment, fracture, and recalcitrant trochanteric bursitis.
- Proximal migration of the osteotomy fragment is rarely a problem since the vastus lateralis prevents significant proximal migration. Similarily, nonunion of the osteotomy is rarely a problem clinically as dense fibrous tissue forms.

■ A fracture of the osteotomy fragment at the vastus tubercle can be problematic, leading to trochanteric escape as subsequent abductor weakness.

Evidence

Aribindi R, Paprosky W, Nourbash P, Kronick J, Barba M. Extended proximal femoral osteotomy. Instr Course Lect. 1999;48:19–26.

The senior author describes the technique of an extended trochanteric osteotomy and reports his early results of 122 patients. In this series, all patients demonstrated union of their osteotomy sites without proximal migration of the osteotomy segment.

Della Valle CJ, Berger RA, Rosenberg AG, Jacobs JJ, Sheinkop MB, Paprosky WG. Extended trochanteric osteotomy in complex primary total hip arthroplasty: a brief note. J Bone Joint Surg [Am]. 2003;85:2385–90.

This study demonstrates how an extended trochanteric osteotomy can be helpful during primary total hip arthroplasty in patients with proximal femoral deformity, developmental hip dysplasia or required hardware removal. Six patients underwent primary hip replacement with an extended trochanteric osteotomy and an extensively coated diaphyseal stem. All patients demonstrated osteointegration.

Masri BA, Campbell DG, Garbuz DS, Duncan CP. Seven specialized exposures for revision hip and knee replacement. Orthop Clin North Am. 1998;29:229–40.

The authors describe how an extended trochanteric osteotomy can be used to facilitate exposure and improve component position in revision total hip replacement.

Paprosky WG, Krishnamurthy A. Five to 14-year follow up on cementless femoral revisions. Orthopedics. 1996;19:765–8.

The senior author describes his mid-term results of using an extensively porous coated implant during femoral revision. The results of 297 hips demonstrated a 2.4% mechanical failure rate at an average of 8 years postoperatively.

Younger TI, Bradford MS, Magnus RE, Paprosky WG. Extended proximal femoral osteotomy: a new technique for femoral revision arthroplasty. J Arthroplasty. 1995;10:329–38.

The senior author describes his initial technique of an extended trochanteric osteotomy. The first 20 patients treated with this technique were reviewed. Excellent cement and component removal and optimal revision component implantation were obtained with no change in postoperative regimen and reliable healing.

Direct Lateral Exposure

Robert B. Bourne

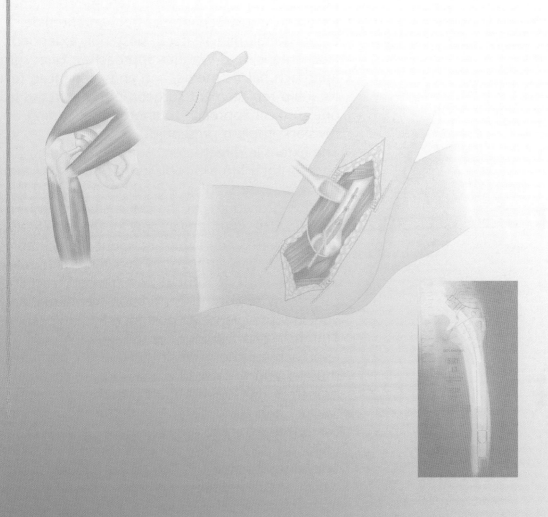

Introduction

- Adequate exposure is considered an essential part of a revision total hip replacement, equal in importance to other steps such as implant extraction dealing with bone defects, implant selection, and postoperative rehabilitation. Many exposures have been described for revision total hip replacement, including transtrochanteric, trochanteric slide, anterolateral, direct lateral, posterior, extended trochanteric, and Wagner approaches. Each surgical approach has its merits, and an experienced revision total hip replacement surgeon often switches from one surgical approach to another depending on the revision problem presented.

- The extensile direct lateral surgical approach for revision total hip arthroplasty has been and remains the workhorse surgical exposure for most of the revision procedures at the University of Western Ontario. The main advantages of the direct lateral approach are wide exposure about the acetabulum and femur, easy conversion to a more extensile approach with or without an extended trochanteric osteotomy or control perforation technique, and a very low prevalence of postoperative dislocations. The main disadvantages of the direct lateral approach are the necessity to split the abductor muscles and the risk of damaging the terminal branch of the superior gluteal nerve.

- Mallory and Head deserve credit for popularizing the use of the extensile direct lateral approach during revision total hip arthroplasties (Head et al., 1987). They also describe the control perforation technique, which enables retained cement to be safely removed from the top of the femur.

- Use of an extended trochanteric osteotomy in association with the extensile direct lateral approach has been popularized by the University of Western Ontario. Like an extended trochanteric osteotomy described through the posterior approach, the lateral bony fragment, which includes the greater trochanter, incorporates approximately one third of the femoral tube and can be extended distally as far as the surgeon needs (usually 10–12 cm).

- The extended trochanteric osteotomy performed through the direct lateral approach is usually hinged on the intermuscular septum. The advantage is that a healthy blood supply is maintained to the bony fragment, but the disadvantage is that the lateral bony fragment and greater trochanter cannot be reflected superiorly.

■ When an extended trochanteric osteotomy is used with the direct lateral approach, the surgeon is usually forced to depend on diaphyseal fixation, and most often an extensively coated cylindrical revision stem is used. At the end of the procedure, two to three cables are used to fix the trochanteric osteotomy fragment to the proximal femur. The surgeon may or may not elect to use one or two strut allografts at this time.

Indications

■ Extensile exposure for revision total hip replacement in patients in whom postoperative dislocation is a risk factor

Examination/Imaging

■ Radiographs should include an anteroposterior view of the pelvis and lateral view of the affected hip, and anteroposterior and lateral views of the affected femur.

■ Judet views are helpful in determining the extent of acetabular osteolysis and whether a pelvic dissociation is present.

■ Computed tomography scans are helpful in assessing the extent of acetabular osteolysis and remaining bone stock.

■ Hip aspiration and the use of a cell count and aerobic and anaerobic cultures are helpful, particularly if the sedimentation rate and C-reactive protein levels are elevated.

PITFALLS

• *Injury to the terminal branch of the superior gluteal nerve, particularly when a major acetabular revision procedure is being performed*

Controversies

• Risk of injury to the terminal branch of the superior gluteal nerve
• Increased risk of postoperative limp and the need for walking aids

Treatment Options

• Anterolateral (Watson-Jones) surgical approach (difficult)
• Posterior surgical approach (associated with high dislocation rates)
• Transtrochanteric surgical approach (risk of trochanteric nonunion/discomfort)
• Extended trochanteric osteotomy through posterior or direct lateral approaches (extensile)
• Extensile direct lateral surgical approach with or without controlled anterior femoral perforations or extended trochanteric osteotomy (extensile)

Surgical Anatomy

- The terminal branch of the superior gluteal nerve courses from posterior to anterior in the interval between the gluteus medius and minimus muscles. The nerve is found 9 cm posteriorly and 5 cm anteriorly from the tip of the greater trochanter (Fig. 1).

- In revision total hip replacement, a posterior longitudinal split in the muscle fibers of the gluteus medius muscle is recommended to avoid the terminal branch of the superior gluteal nerve (Fig. 2). The superior gluteal nerve can be protected by gently retracting the nerve superiorly within the fat layer that exists between the gluteus medius and minimus muscles.

- The anterior portion of the extensor mechanism, including the conjoint tendon of the gluteus medius and gluteus minimus and hip capsule, is then reflected from the anterior aspect of the greater trochanter, maintaining a 5-mm cuff of soft tissue on the anterior aspect of the greater trochanter (Fig. 3). The continuity of the gluteus medius and vastus lateralis muscles is preserved.

- The dissection is then continued distally and posteriorly through the vastus lateralis muscle, thereby avoiding denervating the vastus lateralis and bleeding associated with cutting perforating vessels, which might retract through the intermuscular septum.

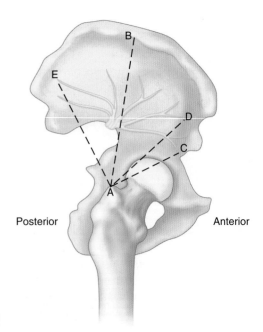

Posterior   Anterior

FIGURE 1

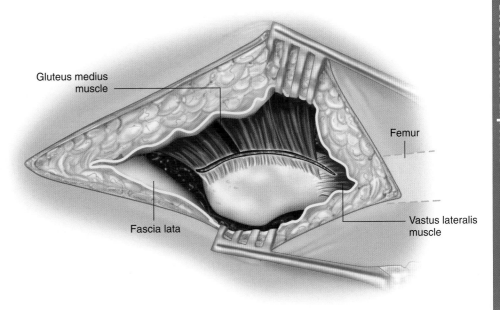

Gluteus medius
muscle

Femur

Fascia lata

Vastus lateralis
muscle

FIGURE 2

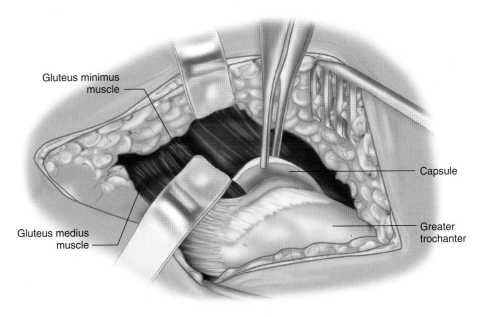

Gluteus minimus
muscle

Capsule

Gluteus medius
muscle

Greater
trochanter

FIGURE 3

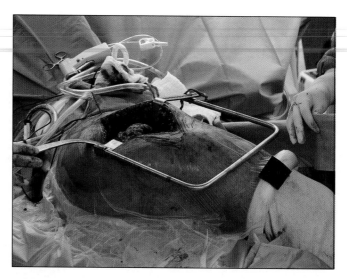

FIGURE 4

Equipment

- Padded operating room table
- Sacral and symphysis bolsters
- Optional anterior and posterior chest bolsters

Positioning

- The patient is positioned in the lateral position on a well-padded operating room table and secured with bolsters.
- The contralateral limb is placed in a slightly flexed position with extra padding placed to protect the common peroneal nerve.
- Padding is placed on the thigh and lower leg, but it is important to keep the contralateral foot and knee palpable through the drapes such that leg-to-leg assessments can be made for final leg length restoration.

Portals/Exposures

- Preexisting hip incisions are usually incorporated into a longitudinal incision in line with the longitudinal axis of the femur and extending one hand breadth proximal to the tip of the greater trochanter and distally as far as is needed for the revision procedure.
- The extensile direct lateral approach is applicable to over 90% of revision hip operations. With extensive acetabular reconstructions (i.e., allografts or use of reconstruction cages). Other surgical approaches (i.e., trochanteric slide or extended trochanteric osteotomy) might be considered to protect the terminal branch of the superior gluteal nerve.

Instrumentation

- The operative procedure is facilitated by the use of self-retaining and Charnley retractors (see Fig. 4).

Controversies

- The advantage of the direct lateral surgical approach for revision total hip arthroplasties is the postoperative stability afforded to these difficult procedures (<0.5% dislocation rates). This must be balanced with the risk of damaging the superior gluteal nerve and subsequent development of limp and need for walking aids.

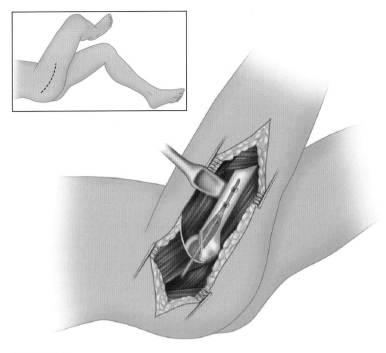

FIGURE 5

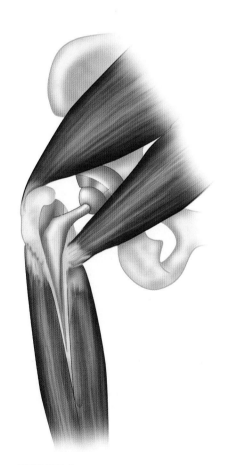

FIGURE 6

PEARLS

- *It is advisable to start the split in the iliotibial band distally, then place a finger between the iliotibial band and greater trochanter to identify the interval between the tensor and gluteus maximus muscles.*

PITFALLS

- *Failure to mobilize the anterior and posterior flaps of the iliotibial band will make the procedure more difficult.*

Instrumentation/ Implantation

- The mobilized iliotibial band can then be reflected using a Charnley retractor.

PEARLS

- *The steps outlined are important to preserve the integrity of the terminal branch of the superior gluteal nerve.*

- *Leaving a 5-mm cuff of soft tissue attached to the anterior aspect of the greater trochanter helps assure an excellent wound closure.*

PITFALLS

- *Making the vertical split in the abductor muscles too anterior can hinder exposure of the proximal femur and result in excessive abductor muscle damage.*

Procedure

STEP 1

- The incision is carried down through the subcutaneous tissue to the iliotibial band, which is then split longitudinally over the femur and carried proximally in the interval between the tensor and gluteus maximus muscles.
- The iliotibial band is mobilized anteriorly and posteriorly, releasing scarring to underlying structures.

STEP 2

- Many variances of the direct lateral approach have been described, but for revision total hip replacements, longitudinally splitting the gluteus medius muscle at the junction of the anterior two thirds and posterior one third as described by Hardinge (1982) is preferred to maximize the safe zone in terms of protecting the terminal branch of the superior gluteal nerve (see Fig. 2).
- The incision is then carried along the anterior aspect of the greater trochanter, leaving a 5-mm cuff of the conjoint tendon for subsequent reattachment to the greater trochanter (see Fig. 3).
- The incision is then carried distal to the greater trochanter and courses posteriorly to preserve the innervation of the vastus lateralis muscle for whatever distance the surgeon requires.
- Once the exposure is outlined, retractors are used to open the vertical split in the gluteus medius muscle and a Cobb elevator used to gently tease fat and the terminal branch of the superior gluteal nerve vascular bundle superiorly off the tendon of the gluteus minimus.
- The visualized gluteus minimus tendon is then split in line with its fibers in the direction of the original incision.
- The conjoint tendinous insertion of the gluteus medius, gluteus minimus, and hip capsule are then reflected anteriorly off the anterior aspect of the greater trochanter, and this exposure is extended distally, elevating the vastus lateralis off the anterolateral femur (Fig. 7).
- Scar and granuloma tissue are then excised, exposing the acetabular and femoral components.
- The goal is to obtain circumferential exposure of the acetabular component and complete exposure of the proximal femur except where the abductor muscles attach to the greater trochanter.

Instrumentation/ Implantation

- Once the anterior flap, consisting of the gluteus medius, gluteus minimus, and hip capsule, is developed, it is helpful to readjust the Charnley retractor, placing a deep blade deep to the anterior abductor cuff of tissue.

Controversies

- Revision total hip replacement requires wider exposure, placing the terminal branch of the superior gluteal nerve at risk. While this complication is largely avoidable, the surgeon might want to consider other options when extensive acetabular revision procedures are needed (i.e., use of allografts or use of a reconstruction cage).

PEARLS

- *Removing cement from the top or using the control perforation technique is ideal if the surgeon wishes to use a cemented or impaction grafting technique for the revision of the femoral component.*

- *Use of an extended trochanteric osteotomy is usually associated with the use of a distal fixation, cementless stem.*

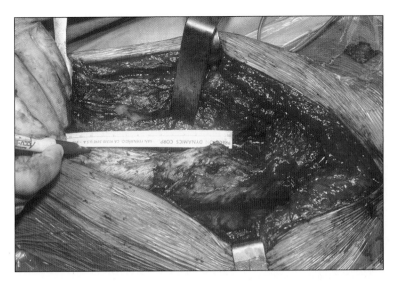

FIGURE 7

STEP 3

- When revising a cemented femoral component from the top, it is advisable to remove the femoral component, then use cement-removing instruments to break the cement away from the underlying bone.
  - It is important to visualize the anterior cortex of the femur to help direct the use of the cement-removing instruments. If visualization becomes difficult, a controlled perforation technique is helpful. A high-speed burr can be used to make 5- to 10-mm circular perforations in the anterior cortex, allowing illumination of the femoral canal and direct visualization of the cement-bone interface. Often, two to three anterior perforations are necessary.
  - When this technique is used, the final femoral stem should be at least two femoral diameters distal to the last perforation to minimize the stress riser effect.

PITFALLS

- *When removing cement from the top, the risk of femoral perforation is increased.*

- *Both the control perforation and extended trochanteric osteotomy techniques necessitate the use of implants that bypass iatrogenic bone defects. Usually these bone defects should be bypassed by at least two cortical diameters or approximately 5 cm.*

Instrumentation/ Implantation

- Specially designed cement removal instruments.

Controversies

- Extended trochanteric osteotomy was first advocated from a posterior surgical approach. Using an extended trochanteric osteotomy from the direct lateral approach is novel. It is important to preserve the vascularity of the trochanteric fragment via attachment of the abductor muscles and the blood supply in the region of the intermuscular septum.

- An alternate measure to improve access to the femoral canal is to develop an extended trochanteric osteotomy through the direct lateral approach.
  - The technique involves making an osteotomy of the posterolateral third of the proximal femur 10 to 15 cm from the tip of the greater trochanter such that the intermuscular septum remains attached to the osteotomy fragment. It is helpful to use a high-speed burr to complete the transverse portion of the osteotomy distally.
  - Use of a ¼-inch osteotome to complete the posterior osteotomy is helpful. The osteotomy is then pried open with the help of a broad osteotome.
  - Wide exposure is obtained using this technique (Fig. 8).

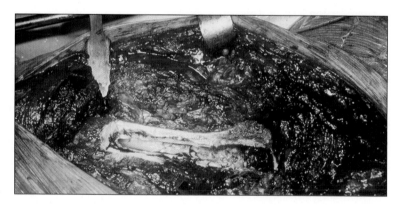

FIGURE 8

STEP 4

- Once the revision procedure has been completed and the surgeon is happy with the stability of the joint and restoration of leg length and offset, closure is begun.
- I prefer to close the vertical incision made in the gluteus minimus tendon with a running 0 PDS (polydioxone) suture.
- The conjoint insertion of the gluteus medius and gluteus minimus and hip capsule are then reapproximated to the cuff of tissue left attached to the anterior aspect of the greater trochanter with interrupted #1 PDS suture. Interrupted sutures are used to close the vertical rent in the gluteus medius muscle belly (Fig. 9). A running #1 PDS suture is used to close the fascia overlying the vastus lateralis muscle.
- The iliotibial band, subcutaneous tissue, and skin are then closed in the usual fashion.

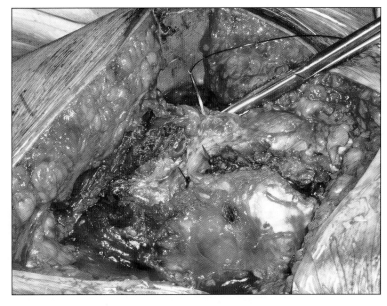

FIGURE 9

Controversies

• Limp is more common after all revision hip arthroplasties related to leg length inequality, abductor muscle weakness, and suboptimal restoration of hip biomechanics. Controversy exists as to whether the extensile direct lateral approach is associated with increased limp as compared to other surgical approaches.

• Controversy also exists as to whether the extensile direct lateral approach is associated with more patients who need walking aids following its use. No proper randomized clinical trial has been performed on this topic.

• It seems evident that the risk of dislocation is at least 10-fold less with the use of the direct lateral approach as compared to posterior surgical approaches during revision, but again, the data are less than ideal in this regard.

Postoperative Care and Expected Outcomes

■ A benefit of the extensile direct lateral approach for revision arthroplasty is the very low risk of postoperative dislocation (<0.5%). Therefore, postoperative precautions to prevent dislocation are minimal (i.e., avoiding flexion over 90° and forced internal rotation for the first 6 weeks).

■ Most revision patients are allowed weight bearing as tolerated depending on stability of the revision reconstruction.

■ Patients are discouraged from performing resisted hip abductor exercises for the first 6 weeks.

■ Most patients prefer to use crutches, and occasionally a walker, if unstable in their gait for the first 3–4 weeks following this type of revision procedure.

Evidence

Baker AS, Bitouris VC. Abductor function after total hip replacement: an electromyelographic and clinical review. J Bone Joint Surg [Br]. 1985;71:47.

A clinical and electromyelographic review of abductor function after use of the direct lateral surgical approach in total hip arthroplasty.

Bauer R, Kerschbaumer F, Poisal S. The transgluteal approach to the hip. Arch Orthop Traumat Surg. 1957;95:47.

A description of one of the variants of the direct lateral surgical approach in total hip arthroplasty.

Demos HA, Rorabeck CH, Bourne RB, MacDonald SJ, McCalden RW. Instability in primary total hip arthroplasty with the direct lateral approach. Clin Orthop Relat Res. 2001;(393):168–80.

A study from our center demonstrating the low risk of dislocation after total hip replacement using the direct lateral surgical approach.

Foster DE, Hunter JR. The direct lateral approach to the hip for arthroplasty: advantages and complications. Orthopaedics. 1987;10:274.

Outline of the advantages and disadvantages of the direct lateral surgical approach during total hip arthroplasty.

Frndak PA, Mallory TH. Translateral surgical approaches to the hip: abductor muscle split. Clin Orthop Relat Res. 1993;(295):135–41.

A description of a variant of the direct lateral hip approach developed by Mallory and Head for total hip replacement.

Hardy AE, Synek V. Hip abductor function after the Hardinge approach: brief report. J Bone Joint Surg [Br]. 1988;70:673.

A review of hip function after total hip replacement using the direct lateral surgical approach.

Hardinge K. The direct lateral approach to the hip. J Bone Joint Surg [Br]. 1982;64: 17–19.

One of the most influential publications supporting use of the direct lateral surgical approach for total hip replacement.

Head WC, Mallory TH, Berklachich FM, Dennis DA, Emerson RH Jr, Wapner KL. Extensile exposure of the hip for revision arthroplasty. J Arthroplasty. 1987;2:265–73.

An important publication outlining the technique of expanding the direct lateral approach to an extensile exposure for revision total hip replacement procedures and using the controlled anterior perforation technique to aid in removing retained cement "from the top".

Jacobs LGH, Buxton RA. The course of the superior gluteal nerve in the lateral approach to the hip. J Bone Joint Surg [Am]. 1989;71:1235.

A study outlining the course of the superior gluteal nerve in the direct lateral approach to the hip.

MacDonald SJ, Cole C, Guerin J, Rorabeck CH, Bourne RB, McCalden RW. Extended trochanteric osteotomy via the direct lateral approach in revision hip arthroplasty. Clin Arthrop. 2003;417:210–16.

Our study outlining the technique and clinical results of combining an extended trochanteric osteotomy with the direct lateral surgical approach during revision total hip replacement.

McFarland B, Osborne G. Approach to the hip: a suggested improvement on Kocher's method. J Bone Joint Surg [Br]. 1954;36:364.

An early publication outlining a variant of the direct lateral approach to the hip.

McLaughlan J. The Stracathro approach to the hip. J Bone Joint Surg [Br]. 1984;66:30.

A paper outlining the so-called "Stracathro" direct lateral approach to the hip.

Minns RJ, Crawford RJ, Porther ML, Hardinge K. Muscle strength following total hip arthroplasty: a comparison of the trochanteric osteotomy and the direct lateral approach. J Arthroplasty. 1993;8:625.

A comparative study comparing the direct lateral and transtrochanteric surgical approaches in total hip arthroplasty, demonstrating at least equivalent abductor strengths in these two patient groups.

Moskal J, Mann JW. A modified direct lateral approach for primary and revision total hip arthroplasty. J Arthroplasty. 1996;11:255–66.

A study promoting use of the direct lateral surgical approach in both primary and revision hip replacement.

Mulliken BD, Rorabeck CH, Bourne RB, Nayak N. A modified direct lateral approach in total hip arthroplasty: a comprehensive review. J Arthroplasty. 1998;13:737–47.

A study demonstrating the modification of the direct lateral surgical approach to the hip used in our center.

Nazarian S, Tesserand PH, Brunet CH. Anatomic basis of the transgluteal approach to the hip. Surg Radiol Anat. 1987;9:27.

A study demonstrating the anatomical rationale of the direct lateral surgical approach to the hip.

Peters PC Jr, Head WC, Emerson RH. An extended trochanteric osteotomy for revision total hip replacement. J Bone Joint Surg [Br]. 1993;75:158–9.

A publication describing the effectiveness of combining a direct lateral surgical approach and extended trochanteric osteotomy during revision total hip replacement.

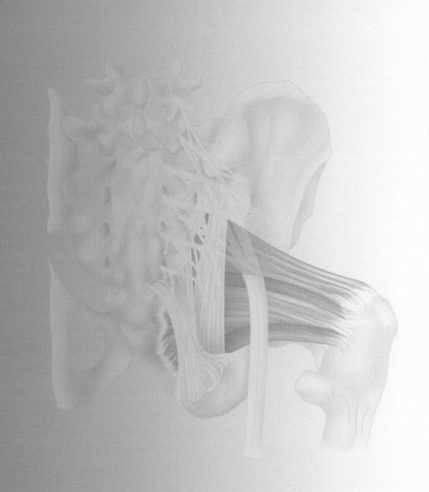

REVISION TOTAL HIP ARTHROPLASTY: TECHNIQUE

Acetabular Cementless Revision

Winston Y. Kim and Bassam A. Masri

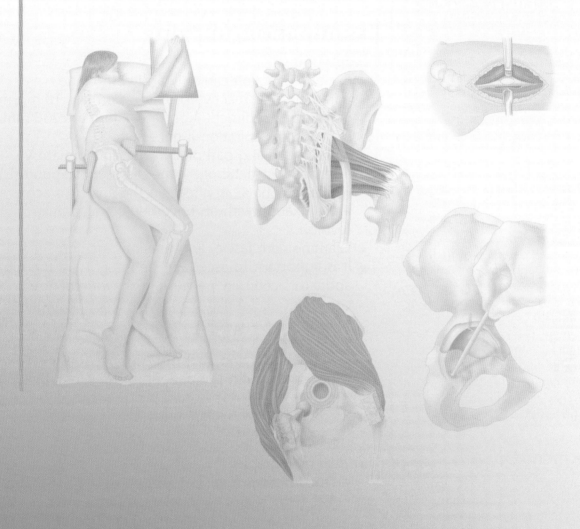

Controversies

- Cementless acetabular reconstruction may be used in small to moderate uncontained (segmental) defects provided adequate peripheral acetabular rim (70–80% intact rim) remains to provide support for the implant.
- Placement of a cementless acetabular implant in a "high" hip center in moderate to severe combined segmental or cavitary defect remains controversial.

Treatment Options

- Cemented acetabular revision in combination with impaction bone grafting in contained bone defects or combined with a reconstruction cage and bone grafting in uncontained/ segmental defects
- Liner exchange with or without bone grafting in a well-fixed acetabular component with pelvic osteolysis
- Cementing a new liner in a well-fixed acetabular component with pelvic osteolysis if the acetabular shell is nonmodular or has a poor locking mechanism

Indications

- Aseptic loosening
- Periprosthetic osteolysis associated with particulate wear debris
- Hip instability secondary to component malposition or soft tissue insufficiency (e.g., abductor dysfunction)
- Hip reimplantation after periprosthetic infection

Examination/Imaging

EXAMINATION

- Exclude infection clinically and with blood parameters (C-reactive protein—normal <10 mg/mL, erythrocyte sedimentation rate—normal <230 mm/hr) and hip aspiration if necessary.
- Note underlying pathology (e.g., inflammatory arthropathy, metabolic bone disease, osteoporosis), which may have an effect on the ability to achieve initial fixation with an uncemented acetabular revision.
- Examine skin, fascia, and previous incisions.
- It is important to ascertain the integrity of the hip abductors clinically because, if they are deficient, a constraint acetabular component may be required.
  - Trendelenburg test
  - Palpation
  - Active abduction against resistance; best performed with the patient in the lateral decubitus position
- Examine neurovascular status.

IMAGING

- Plain radiographs
  - Obtain pelvis (Fig. 1A), obturator (Fig. 1B), and iliac (Fig. 1C) oblique views; anteroposterior (AP) and lateral views of the hip (Fig. 2); and AP and lateral full-length femur views.
  - Evaluate extent of bone loss.
  - Previous radiographs are useful to assess progression of osteolytic lesion and implant migration or subsidence.
- Previous operative notes and manufacturers' implant labels must be obtained prior to surgery.
- Computed tomography (CT) scanning is rarely required or useful due to artifacts from preexisting implants; however, if pelvic discontinuity is suspected, CT reconstruction images may be helpful in demonstrating the extent of structural integrity.

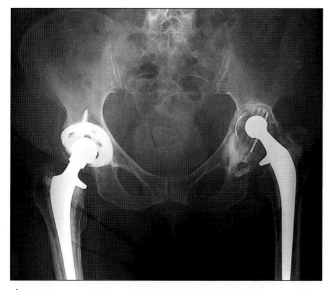

A

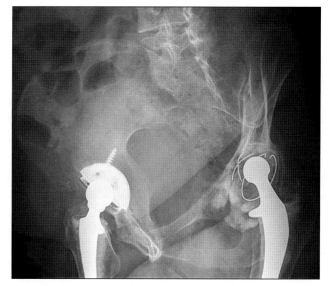

B

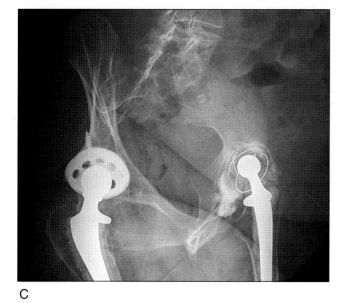

C

FIGURE 1

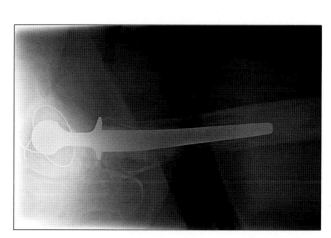

FIGURE 2

Surgical Anatomy

- The sciatic nerve is the key structure at risk during revision arthroplasty (Fig. 3).
  - The nerve can be identified by rolling it under the surgeon's finger as it crosses the ischium posterior to the acetabulum; this allows the surgeon to avoid retractor injury.
  - The sciatic nerve emerges deep and inferior to the piriformis and superficial to the obturator internus and gemelli.
- The "safe zone" for insertion of acetabular screws is the posterior superior quadrant of the acetabulum (Fig. 4). Screw insertion in this zone minimizes the risk of catastrophic vascular injury.

Positioning

- The patient is placed in the lateral decubitus position, ensuring a vertical pelvis.
- Pressure areas are padded to protect skin and neurovascular structures.
- During positioning, place the lower limb in the position in which acetabular preparation would occur when securing the pelvis. For example, with a posterior approach, the pelvis tends to tilt anteriorly when the femur is retracted anteriorly in the course of acetabular exposure. This should be compensated for when positioning at the beginning of the procedure.

PEARLS

- *Make sure that the pelvis is stable, and that the final position of the pelvis after retraction is known. This is done by applying forward (for posterior approach) or backward (for lateral approach) pressure to the femur when positioning in the lateral decubitus position. The pelvis should be vertical with the simulated retraction on the femur.*

PITFALLS

- *Ensure that patient positioning is performed under surgeon supervision, as inaccurate positioning or loss of position during surgery may lead to errors during acetabular preparation (e.g., excessive reaming of posterior column) or errors in component alignment.*

Equipment

- Any appropriate positioning device may be used, provided the pelvis is held secure throughout the procedure.

Controversies

- Some surgeons prefer the supine position for the lateral approach; however, most surgeons in North America prefer the lateral decubitus position.

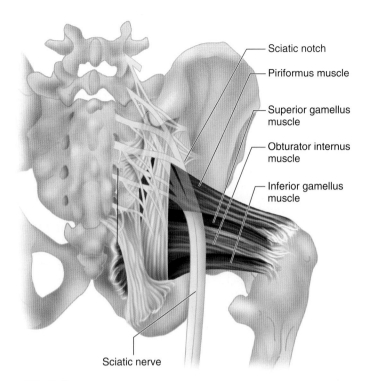

Sciatic notch

Piriformus muscle

Superior gamellus muscle

Obturator internus muscle

Inferior gamellus muscle

Sciatic nerve

FIGURE 3

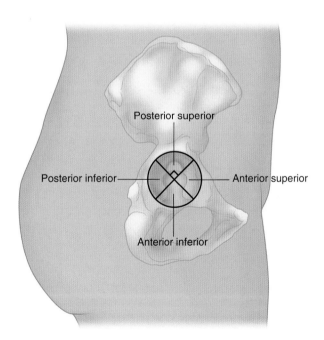

Posterior superior

Posterior inferior

Anterior superior

Anterior inferior

FIGURE 4

Portals/Exposures

- The surgical approach is chosen after careful preoperative consideration of clinical and radiographic factors.
  - Clinical factors
    - Patient anatomy
    - Previous approach
    - Isolated or both component revision
    - Potential for hip instability
    - Abductor function
    - Surgeon preference and training
  - Radiographic factors
    - Extent and anticipated region of bone loss
    - Presence of pelvic discontinuity
- The options are:
  - Direct lateral
  - Posterolateral
  - Trochanteric osteotomy
  - Trochanteric slide (flip) osteotomy
  - Extended trochanteric osteotomy

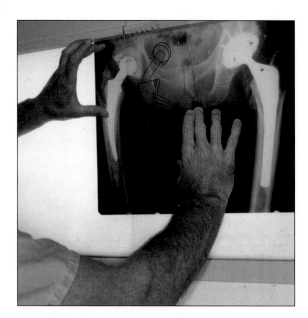

FIGURE 5

Instrumentation

- The use of an elevated, padded stand placed at the foot of the patient allows placement of the operative limb in an abducted, internally rotated, and extended position during the posterolateral approach, which facilitates exposure of the short external rotators and protects the sciatic nerve.

Procedure

STEP 1: SURGICAL EXPOSURE AND REMOVAL OF COMPONENTS

- Ensure optimal surgical exposure prior to attempting removal of acetabular components.
- Care must be taken to ensure no further bone loss.
- Identify the interface between implant and bone with use of rongeur, cautery, osteotomes, and metal-tipped burrs.
- Remove a well-fixed component with curved osteotomes or a system of curved osteotomes (i.e., the Explant system) (Fig. 6).
  - The Explant system consists of a rotating handle connected to a central femoral head and a curved osteotome that inserts into preexisting or trial liner.
  - Two curved osteotomes are used sequentially, beginning with a short blade, which creates a channel, followed by a second full-radius blade.
- Perform careful and thorough débridement of all fibrous and membranous tissue with a Cobb elevator, a rongeur, metal-tipped burrs, or cautery prior to assessment of remaining bone stock.

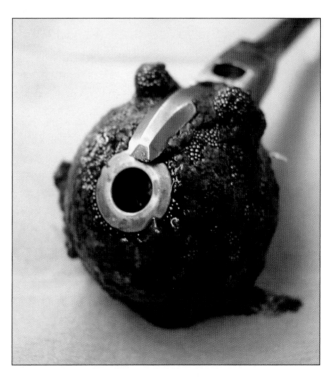

FIGURE 6

PEARLS

- *Successful revision with a cementless component requires adequate bony support in the dome, posterior column, and inferior portion of the acetabulum. The anterior column is of little importance. Any cavitary or medial defects should be grafted.*

- *Avoid excessive reaming of the posterior column. If necessary, the anterior column may be sacrificed to protect the posterior column.*

STEP 2: CLASSIFICATION OF REMAINING ACETABULAR BONE STOCK

- The optimal acetabular reconstruction is determined by the extent and location of bone loss and quality of remaining host bone.
- Assess integrity of the supportive rim to determine if any bone defect is contained (cavitary defect) or uncontained (segmental defect) (Fig. 7).
- A useful and widely employed classification of acetabular defects is the Paprosky classification.
  - Type 1: acetabular rim and wall/dome intact; columns intact and supportive
  - Type 2: distortion of acetabular rim and dome/wall; columns intact and supportive
  - Type 3: absent acetabular rim; wall/dome and columns compromised
- Cementless acetabular revision with a hemispherical porous coated shell is optimal in Paprosky type 1 acetabular defects (Fig. 8).
- In type 2 defects, restoration of the distorted wall or dome with bone grafting (particulate or structural) or augments are necessary prior to cementless acetabular reconstruction.
- Paprosky type 3 acetabular defects require fixation and restoration of the columns with a reconstruction plate prior to acetabular reconstruction (Fig. 9).

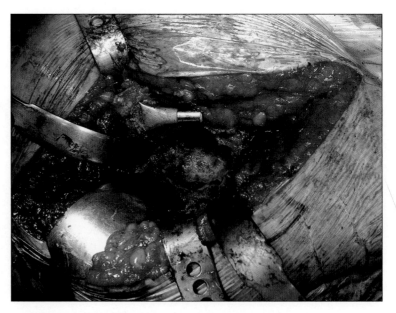

FIGURE 7

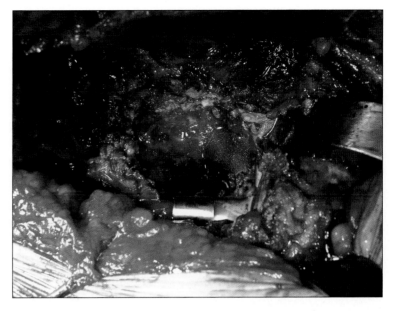

FIGURE 8

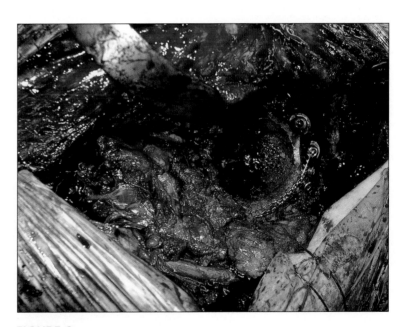

FIGURE 9

Instrumentation/ Implantation

- Screw fixation should take into account the "safe zone" for screw insertion to avoid neurovascular injury.

STEP 3: RECONSTRUCTION WITH CEMENTLESS ACETABULAR IMPLANT

- The vast majority of acetabular revisions may be performed using a hemispherical uncemented acetabular cup.
- The acetabulum is progressively reamed in 1- to 2-mm increments to expose bleeding host bone, hemispheric surface, and an intact peripheral rim (Fig. 10).
- Small contained (cavitary) defects are filled with autograft or particulate allograft. Reverse reaming of the graft ensures that the allograft or autograft is impacted and pressurized.
- Press-fit an appropriate implant 2 mm larger than the last reamer utilized.
- Confirm optimal alignment both of lateral opening and anteversion using an external alignment jig.
- Ensure that the acetabular component is uniformly in contact with the underlying host bone ("bottomed out") by using a fine-tipped suction through perforations in the acetabular shell.
- Supplementary screw fixation is almost always necessary in revision surgery (Fig. 11).
- The appropriate-sized trial or definitive liner is inserted into the shell after satisfactory acetabular fixation is obtained.
- We recommend against use of a 28-mm femoral head if the outside diameter is greater than 62 mm.

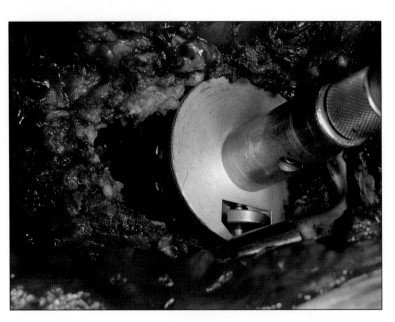

FIGURE 10

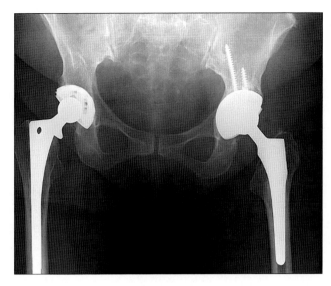

FIGURE 11

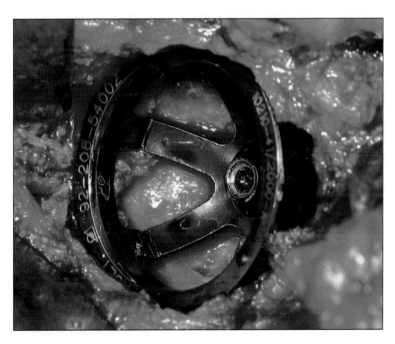

FIGURE 12

Controversies

- Recently developed trabecular metal acetabular shells may be advantageous in achieving more rapid initial stability because of their higher coefficient of friction and higher porosity for bone ingrowth; however, results are preliminary and further long-term evaluation is required.

Regardless, as long as the polyethylene thickness is adequate (>5–6 mm), the largest possible head diameter may be used with a highly cross-linked polyethylene liner.

- If the shell is medialized, an offset liner may be used to restore offset on the acetabular side.
- Similarly, if a jumbo cup is used, the center of rotation may be brought back down to a more normal level by using an eccentric liner.

Complications

- Hip instability and dislocation are the most common complications after revision arthroplasty.
  - The use of large-diameter femoral heads may reduce the risk of postoperative hip instability.
  - Extended lip liners and constraint liners should be available if required, in appropriate patients.
  - Skirted modular heads should be avoided if possible because of the risk of impingement and dislocation.
- The risks of periprosthetic infection are higher than in primary arthroplasty.
- Judicious placement of retractors and insertion of acetabular screws with attention to the safe zones of acetabular screw insertion will minimize the risk of neurovascular compromise.

Postoperative Care and Expected Outcomes

- An abduction pillow should be kept between the patient's legs in the immediate postoperative period.
- Most patients are encouraged to ambulate within 24 hours of surgery, with assistance if necessary. We usually allow partial weight bearing, but this can be at the discretion of the surgeon.
- Postoperative care is individualized according to the complexity of the procedure, fixation obtained, and hip stability documented at the time of operation.
- The complexity of revision acetabular arthroplasty varies, and reported results of acetabular aspetic loosening and failure vary according to the complexity of bone loss.

Evidence

Della Valle C, Berger R, Rosemberg A, Galante JO. Cementless acetabular reconstruction in revision total hip arthroplasty. Clin Orthop Relat Res. 2004;(420):96–100.

This study is a retrospective review of 138 cementless acetabular reconstructions with a mean follow-up of 15 years. (Level IV evidence [case series])

Hallstrom BR, Golladay GJ, Vittetoe DA, Harris WH. Cementless acetabular revision with the Harris-Galante porous prosthesis. J Bone Joint Surg [Am]. 2004;86: 1007–100.

This study reviews 122 cementless acetabular hip reconstructions by the senior author with a mean follow-up of 12.5 years. (Level IV evidence [case series])

Mitchell PA, Masri BA, Garbuz DS, Greidanus NV, Wilson D, Duncan CP. Removal of well fixed, cementless, acetabular components in revision hip arthroplasty. J Bone Joint Surg [Br]. 2003;85:949–52.

The authors described in detail a series of 31 hip implants removed using a new cup extraction system. (Level IV evidence [case series])

Paprosky WG, Perona PG, Lawrence JM. Acetabular defect classification and surgical reconstruction in revision arthroplasty: a 6 year follow-up evaluation. J Arthroplasty. 1994;9:33–44.

This study describes in detail the rationale for a system widely used in the classification of acetabular bone deficiency in revision arthroplasty.

Wasielewski RC, Cooperstein LA, Kruger MP, Rubash HE. Acetabular anatomy and the transacetabular fixation of screws in total hip arthroplasty. J Bone Joint Surg [Am]. 1990;72:501–8.

The authors described the quadrant system for safe screw placement through an acetabular component.

Rings and Cages

Catherine F. Kellett, Petros J. Boscainos, and Allan E. Gross

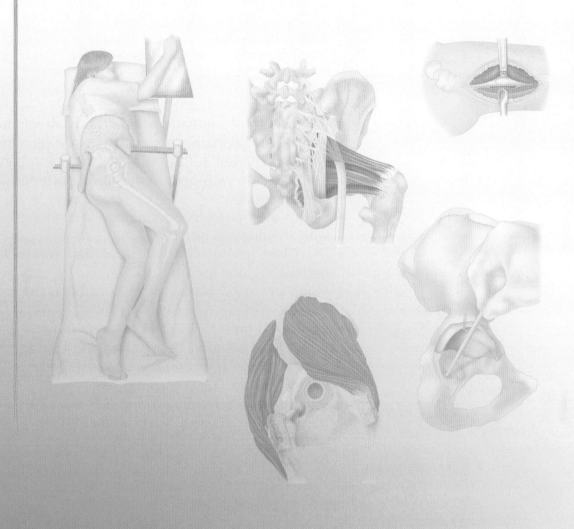

Indications

- There are two types of rings: the roof reinforcement ring and the antiprotrusio (or ilioischial) cage.
  - The roof ring primarily protects the dome of the acetabulum and extends from the ilium superiorly to the inferomedial aspect of the acetabulum.
  - The antiprotrusio cage extends from the ilium superiorly to the ischium, inferiorly spanning and protecting the entire acetabulum.

ROOF RING

- Primary hip replacement
  - Protrusio: posttraumatic osteoarthritis, rheumatoid arthritis, or idiopathic protrusion in combination with morcellized autograft bone, providing contact can be made with host bone superoposteriorly and inferomedially
  - Severe osteoporosis: osteoporosis in conjunction with rheumatoid arthritis
  - Dysplasia: to protect a structural graft and provide better coverage for the cup
- Revision hip arthroplasty with loss of bone stock due to osteolysis
  - Contained defects: in combination with morcellized allograft bone, providing contact can be made with host bone superoposteriorly and inferomedially.
  - Uncontained defects involving less than 50% of the acetabulum: small structural allografts supporting less than 50% of the cup can be protected by a roof ring.

CAGE

- Primary hip replacement
  - Severe protrusion in combination with morcellized autograft bone where the defect is so large that it cannot be spanned by a roof ring
- Revision hip arthroplasty
  - Large contained defects: contained defects involving the entire acetabulum requiring a device that spans from ilium to ischium, used with morcellized allograft bone.
  - Uncontained defects involving more than 50% of the acetabulum. The cage can be used in conjunction with a structural allograft.

- *If a roof ring is used in a massive defect, the ring will be sitting on morsellized bone inferomedially and will toggle and loosen.*

- *The present generation of rings does not achieve biologic fixation by bone ongrowth or ingrowth and really only serve as a buttress plate while the bone graft heals. They therefore have the potential to fail in the mid- to long-term.*

- *Treating large segmental acetabular defects that comprise more than 50% of the acetabulum is one of the most difficult challenges in revision arthroplasty of the hip. One of the surgical options is a structural acetabular allograft. Unless these allografts are protected by a cage that extends from ilium to ischium, there is an unacceptable incidence of graft failure.*

- Pelvic discontinuity: a cage is used to bridge the discontinuity. A graft may also be necessary. If the cage does not stabilize the discontinuity, a plate can be used with the cage.
- The cage has a limited life span, but by facilitating restoration of bone, it allows the next revision at the correct anatomic level with a cementless cup. Therefore, in a younger, higher demand patient, this may be a better choice.
- Cages can be used in irradiated bone and also allow use of a constrained cup.

Controversies

- If a pelvic discontinuity is demonstrated radiologically and intraoperatively, a posterior column plate in addition to the cage should be considered.
- If the bone defect involves greater than 50% of the acetabulum but contact can still be made with the inferomedial part of the host acetabulum, then a roof ring can be used. It must be emphasized, however, that there is a fine line between using an uncemented cup and a roof ring; just by reaming, a little more contact can be made with host bone in order to use an uncemented cup. However, if the contained defect is global, affecting the entire acetabulum, and contact with 50% of the host bone is not possible even with more reaming, and contact with the inferomedial host acetabulum is not possible, then a cage is necessary.
- The roof ring use at the authors' institution has decreased after the introduction of trabecular metal (TM) cups.
- TM cups with augments is another option for many types of defects. The TM cup with augment uses the oblong cup principle (of filling the defect), but since the augment is separate from the cup, one can place the cup independently.
- We use the following algorithm:
  - Low-demand patients—TM cup and augment
  - High-demand patients who may require another revision in their lifetime—TM cup and shelf (minor column) graft

Treatment Options

- Most contained defects can be managed by uncemented cups with good mid- to long-term results (jumbo cups). Cementless cups permit only limited restoration of bone stock. They should not be used in irradiated bone.
- The use of trabecular metal has the potential to reduce the necessary amount of host bone contact. Another alternative is impaction grafting, a technique that involves cementing a cup onto a bed of impacted allograft bone.
- Alternatives to rings and cages are the custom triflanged cup, an oblong cup, a minor column structural graft, or impaction grafting.
- Another controversial solution to acetabular defects is to place the cup in a high and/or protruded position.

Examination/Imaging

- Most bone defects can be defined by routine radiographs. Judet oblique views may be helpful to define the anterior and posterior columns. The final definition of the defect must be made intraoperatively after removal of the old components.
- Classification of bone defects:
  - I—no significant loss of bone
  - II—contained (cavitary) loss of bone where columns and rim are intact
  - III—uncontained (segmental) loss of bone stock involving less than 50% of the acetabulum
  - IV—uncontained loss of bone stock involving greater than 50% of the acetabulum
  - V—pelvic discontinuity with uncontained loss of bone
- Figure 1 shows osteolysis around the acetabular component, suitable for reconstruction with a ring.
- Figure 2 shows massive osteolysis and acetabular component migration, suitable for reconstruction with a cage.

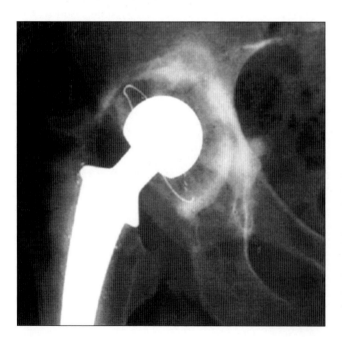

FIGURE 1

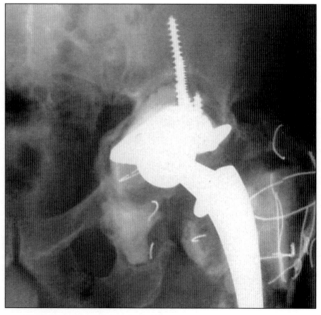

FIGURE 2

Equipment

• Vacuum beanbag or side supports and props
• Armboard and support
• Pillows or gel pad for padding

Positioning

■ Place the patient in the lateral position on the operating table.
■ Secure the patient well with a sandbag or posts.
■ Pad the contralateral knee (peroneal nerve) and pressure points.
■ Give prophylactic antibiotics.

Portals/Exposures

■ Either a posterior or a lateral (transgluteal) approach will give adequate exposure for insertion of a roof ring. Insertion of a cage, however, requires exposure of the ischium.
■ We prefer a trochanteric osteotomy to expose the ischium; however, a posterior approach is also adequate and can be converted to a trochanteric osteotomy if necessary. The trochanteric osteotomy that we prefer is the trochanteric slide because it has a lower incidence of trochanteric escape.
■ A trochanteric slide is carried out through a straight lateral incision.
■ After the fascia lata has been incised, the posterior border of the gluteus medius and minimus is identified and retracted anteriorly (Fig. 3). The vastus lateralis is reflected off the intermuscular septum for 6–8 cm, and reflected anteriorly for 1 or 2 cm.

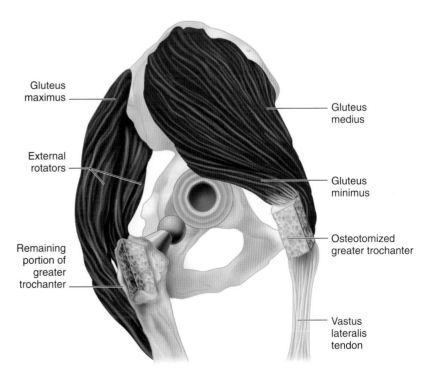

FIGURE 3

- We do not release the external rotators or posterior capsule.
- The trochanteric osteotomy is then carried out using an oscillating saw, with the osteotomy being done posterior to anterior and ending distally about 2 cm distal to the insertion of the vastus lateralis into the vastus ridge (Fig. 4, *dotted line*).
- In order to keep the posterior capsule and external rotators intact, we retain about 1 cm of bone posteriorly, attached to the main femoral fragment. The main trochanteric fragment is retracted anteriorly and an anterior capsulectomy carried out. The hip is dislocated anterolaterally but retracted posteriorly, and the trochanteric fragment anteriorly.
- If more exposure is required, a trochanteric slide can be converted to a transverse trochanteric osteotomy by releasing the vastus off the trochanter so the trochanter can be reflected superiorly. The ischium can also be exposed via an extended trochanteric osteotomy if a difficult femoral implant removal is anticipated.

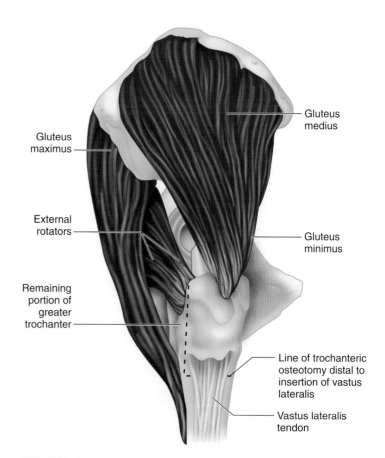

Gluteus maximus

Gluteus medius

External rotators

Gluteus minimus

Remaining portion of greater trochanter

Line of trochanteric osteotomy distal to insertion of vastus lateralis

Vastus lateralis tendon

FIGURE 4

■ The ischium is identified by tracing down the posterior rim of the acetabulum until the ischium is reached. The ischium extends out from the acetabular rim posteroinferiorly and is quite prominent. It can be cleared gently with an elevator for 1 or 2 cm for confirmation. The ligaments that come off the ischium are then encountered. Going beyond this endangers the sciatic nerve.

Procedure

STEP 1

■ After removal of the acetabular implant and the membrane, spherical reaming is carried out. Then a decision is made as to whether a cementless cup, a roof ring, or a cage is going to be used.
  • Using a trial cup, if contact can be made with bleeding host bone over an area of approximately 50%, particularly superiorly and posteriorly, then a cementless cup can be used.
  • If this is not possible but contact with host acetabulum is possible superiorly and inferomedially, then a roof ring can be used.
  • If this is not possible, a cage is necessary.
■ Most of this decision making is done before surgery, but final confirmation is done intraoperatively as described.
■ After removal of the acetabular component and débridement, the defect is defined. The ilium, dome, and anterior and posterior columns are examined.

PEARLS

- *If there is segmental loss of bone posterosuperiorly involving the dome and posterior column so the cup cannot be stabilized at the correct or near-correct anatomic level, then a structural graft is indicated. If the host bone support for the cup is 50–70%, then a minor column (shelf) graft (as already discussed) is indicated, but if the host bone support is less than 50%, a major column graft is indicated.*

PITFALLS

- *Long-term studies show that cages can fail by fracturing of the flanges. This can be avoided by making sure the cage or roof ring is solidly supported by host bone or bone graft.*

Instrumentation/ Implantation

- A separate allograft preparation table is needed to prepare the allograft. This can be done at the same time as the acetabular preparation by one of the surgeon's assistants.

STEP 2: RECONSTRUCTING THE ACETABULUM

- The type of bone defect dictates the method of reconstruction:
  - Type II contained defect—repaired with morcellized graft (Fig. 5A)
  - Type III uncontained shelf defect (<50% of acetabulum)—repaired with structural graft (Fig. 5B)
  - Type IV uncontained defect (>50% of acetabulum)—repaired with structural graft (Fig. 5C)
  - Type V pelvic discontinuity—repaired with structural graft (Fig. 5D)
- The optimal allograft bone for revision is deep-frozen.
- If the defect is contained, then morcellized allograft is used.
  - The fragments should ideally be 5–10 mm in diameter.
  - The morcellized bone is impacted to form a solid base to support the ring or cage. Impaction is carried out using reverse reaming. The diameter of the final reamer determines the outer diameter of the ring to be used.
  - A structural graft may have to be reamed lightly, leaving the subchondral bone intact, in order to accommodate the outer diameter of the ring. When a structural graft is used, any additional cavitary defects are filled with morcellized bone.
  - It is important that the ring is solidly supported by allograft or host bone.
- Acetabular allograft bone is usually used for structural grafts, but a male femoral head shaped to fit the defect is acceptable.

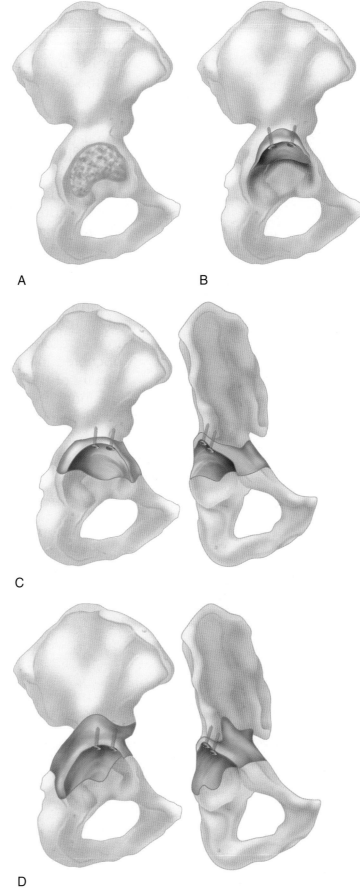

A

B

C

D

FIGURE 5

STEP 3: ROOF RING INSERTION

- After restoration of bone stock, the diameter of the bony bed should match the outer diameter of the roof ring. The outer diameter of the ring corresponds to the last reamer used. Prior to impaction, placement and adjustment by hand may be required.
- Using the cup positioner, impact the roof ring with the flange superiorly and slightly posteriorly (Fig. 6). It should feel solid even before insertion of the screws.
- If a roof ring is used, it must have host bone support superoposteriorly and inferomedially. Make sure it is stable against host bone superiorly, posteriorly, and inferomedially.
- The ring is then fixed by 6.5-mm fully threaded cancellous screws provided with the ring. The screws are inserted through the holes in the superior flange of the ring into the dome of the acetabulum, usually in a vertical to oblique direction, and should be anchored in host bone (Fig. 7). Depending on the quality of the bone, it may be necessary to engage the inner cortex. Insert dome screws in a superior (load-bearing) direction. At least three screws should be used.

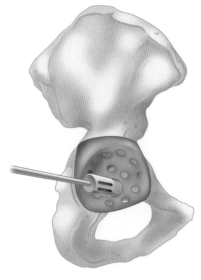

FIGURE 6

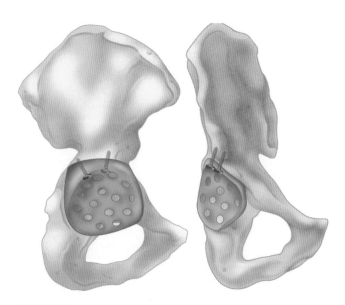

FIGURE 7

STEP 4: CAGE INSERTION

- After restoration of bone stock, the diameter of the bony bed should match the outer diameter of the cage.
- Using trial cages if available, the surgeon can determine the size of the cage and whether or not the flanges need bending in order to make host contact. The outer diameter of the ring should correspond to the last reamer used.
- It may be necessary to contour the flanges to provide a good press fit against host bone.
  - The flanges should only be bent in one direction (avoid reverse bending) or they will be weakened. Normally the upper flanges have to be bent downward toward the ilium and the lower flange slightly upward to accommodate the shape of the ischium.
  - Perform all contouring before inserting the screws so that the cage does not displace as the screws are tightened.
- The muscle is cleared off the ilium to create room for the superior flanges.
- Stabilize the cage in the acetabulum with the superior flanges against the ilium superiorly and slightly posterior.
- The inferior flange may be slotted into the ischium or placed against the ischium. If the flange is placed against the ischium, the cup may end up in a slightly lateral position, so we prefer to slot the cage into the ischium.

- To prepare a slot in the ischium for the implant, first identify the ischium by palpating down the posterior rim of the acetabulum. The site can be confirmed by drilling a 3.2-mm hole in the ischium and checking the position with a depth gauge. The depth gauge should encounter bone circumferentialy to a depth of at least 4 cm in a posteroinferior direction (Fig. 8). A radiograph can be taken to confirm the position. Several small drill holes can be made into the ischium. A small osteotome is then used in a direction parallel to the ischium to initiate the slot.

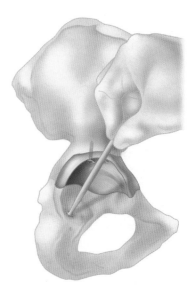

FIGURE 8

- Once the starter slot has been created, the ischial flange of the cage is used to complete the slot.
- Prior to impaction, hand placement can be used if required.
- The cage is impacted with the cup positioner, making sure it is stable against host bone. The ischial flange is inserted first and then the ring is impacted, seating the superior flanges on the ilium.
- Once the cage is firmly seated with the flanges against bone, insert two 6.5-mm fully threaded cancellous screws into the dome (Fig. 9).

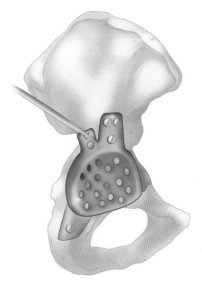

FIGURE 9

Controversies

- Recently the authors have performed several surgeries in which they have combined a TM revision cup and a cage. In this situation we have postulated that the TM cup will provide a better environment for the graft (morcellized or structural), but because of less than optimal host bone contact it has to be protected by a cage. The cage would protect the TM cup until the morcellized graft has remodeled or the structural graft united, and then the stress will be off the cage and on the TM cup. This may prevent early failure of the cage by fracture of the ischial flange.

- Then insert two or three 6.5-mm fully threaded cancellous screws into the superior flanges.
- If the inferior flange had been placed against the ischium, one or two 6.5-mm fully threaded cancellous screws should be inserted inferiorly.
- Depending on the bone quality, it may be necessary for the screws to engage the inner cortex for adequate fixation.
- The inferior flange can be stabilized in three ways. For contained defects, simply buttress the inferior flange against the ischium without screw fixation. For segmental defects and for discontinuity, screw the inferior flange against the ischium with 1 or 2 screws, or slot the flange into the ischium. We prefer the slot technique for contained and uncontained defects.
- It is important to identify and protect the sciatic nerve, especially if screwing the flange against the ischium.

PEARLS

- *Cups are cemented into rings, allowing adjustment of version independent of the ring and the local delivery of antibiotics.*

- *Prior to cementing the cup, a trial reduction to evaluate cup position must be carried out.*

- *Leg length is also evaluated using a reference outrigger guide inserted into the iliac crest during exposure.*

PITFALLS

- *Dislocations can be avoided by orienting the cup independently of the position of the ring. In the multiply operated hip with poor abductor function, a constrained cup can be cemented into the ring. Another preventive measure is the use of a brace for 3 months following surgery.*

STEP 5

- An all-polyethylene cup is cemented into the roof ring or cage.
- Use the cup trials to determine which size to use. Aim to allow for a uniform 3-mm cement mantle.
- It is important to orient the cup independently of the roof ring or cage, using the same landmarks as if the cup were inserted directly into the acetabulum.
- Prepare the cement and pack it into the roof ring or cage once it is in its doughy state (Fig. 10).
- Assemble the cup onto the alignment guide and insert the cup into the cement (Fig. 11).
- The cup should be inclined at approximately 45° with 20° of anteversion, independent of the roof ring or cage orientation. It is important to cement the cup in the correct anatomic position regardless of the position of the ring. If indicated, a snap-in or constrained cup can be cemented into a ring.
- Maintain pressure on the cup and cement until the cement has hardened. Some cement penetrates the holes in the ring and reaches the surface of the structural allograft or the surface of the impacted allograft bone. Trim off the excess cement.

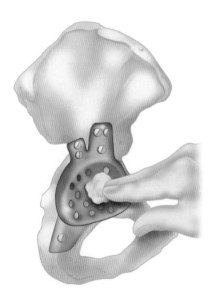

FIGURE 10

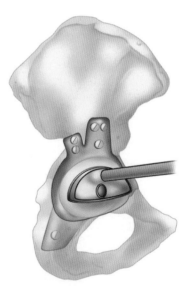

FIGURE 11

Step 6

- The greater trochanter is reattached with two 16-gauge cerclage wires passed inferior to the lesser trochanter.
- The rest of the closure is routine.
- Figure 12 shows a postoperative radiograph of reconstruction with a ring.
- Figure 13 shows a postoperative radiograph of reconstruction with a cage.

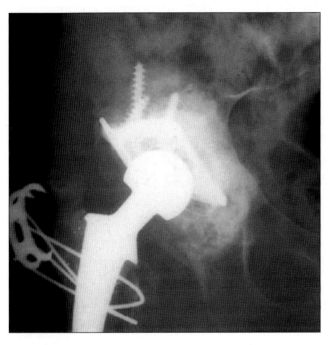

FIGURE 12

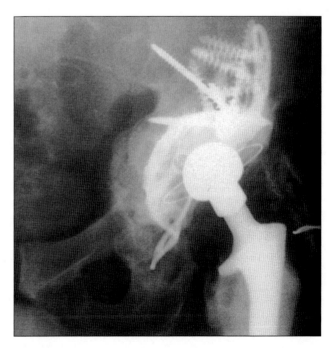

FIGURE 13

Postoperative Care and Expected Outcomes

- Routine antibiotic and deep venous thrombosis prophylaxis are used.
- Postoperative weight-bearing status depends on the type and magnitude of bone grafting and what the patient will tolerate.
  - When the roof ring is used with morcellized bone graft, the patient can bear weight as tolerated.
  - When the roof ring is used to protect a small structural graft, weight bearing should be delayed for 3 months (kept featherweight bearing for 6 weeks and then partial weight bearing at 60–80 lbs for 6 weeks).
  - When the cage is used to protect a graft, morcellized or structural, weight bearing should also be delayed for 3 months (kept featherweight bearing for 6 weeks and then partial weight bearing at 60–80 lbs for 6 weeks).
- Gentle passive range-of-motion exercises are started at 2–3 days with no flexion beyond 70° and no adduction.
- Active abduction in the supine position is allowed at 6 weeks and against gravity at 12 weeks to protect the trochanteric repair.
- The midterm (5–10 years) results should be at least 75% successful with re-revision rates of 10–20%, keeping in mind that these are revisions considered beyond the scope of uncemented cups.
- Most authors agree that the use of rings and bone grafting facilitates the next revision.

OUTCOMES

- Using morcellized bone protected by a roof ring for contained acetabular defects, at an average follow-up of 5 years in 43 hips there was 1 re-revision, with an additional 4 hips with asymptomatic loosening. For uncontained defects involving greater than 50% of the acetabulum in eight patients in whom a major column structural allograft was used in conjunction with a cage, at an average follow-up of 7.5 years there was one failure due to infection (Saleh et al., 2000).
- In a later paper, we reported on 13 patients with an average follow-up of 10.5 years with clinical and radiographic success in 10 hips (77%) (Saleh et al., 2000). In a later study of cages, there were six patients with sciatic nerve injuries, all of whom made

Complications

- The most common complication related to the present generation of rings is loss of fixation. In our series (Goodman et al., 2004), four rings lost fixation, all requiring revision, and another three had fractured flanges. This problem relates to the fact that the present generation of rings does not achieve biologic fixation, and the rings really only serve as a buttress plate while the bone graft heals. If and when the ring fails, the bone graft may have incorporated enough to restore bone stock for an uncemented cup. Any motion between the ring and host or grafted bone will eventually cause the ring to loosen or fracture. The rings are going to have to be made of a material that achieves biologic fixation and provides a friendly environment for bone healing (i.e., TM).

significant partial or full recovery. All six cases were associated with placing the inferior flange on top of the ischium rather than slotting it inside the ischium. Three rings had fractured flanges, one of which was revised. This can be avoided by making sure the ring is solidly supported by host bone or bone graft. Seven hips dislocated (11%); this can be avoided by orienting the cup independently of the position of the ring (Goodman et al., 2004). Also, in the multiply operated hip with poor abductor function, a constrained cup can be cemented into the ring. Another preventive measure is the use of a brace for 3 months following surgery.

Evidence

Berry DJ. Antiprotrusio cages for acetabular revision. Clin Orthop Relat Res. 2004;(420):106–12.

Wide exposure of the acetabulum, positioning the cage to span host bone–to–host bone bridging defects, and secure fixation of the cage with a good dome and posterior column support are recommended.

Berry DJ, Lewallen DG, Hanssen AD, Cabanela ME. Pelvic discontinuity in revision total hip arthroplasty. J Bone Joint Surg [Am]. 1999;81:1692–702.

Pelvic discontinuity is uncommon, and treatment is associated with a high rate of complications. For hips with type IVa bone loss and selected hips with type IVb defects, in which a socket inserted without cement can be satisfactorily supported by native bone, we prefer to use a posterior column plate to stabilize the pelvis and a porous-coated socket inserted without cement. For most hips with type IVb and type IVc bone loss, we prefer to use particulate bone graft or a single structural bone graft protected with an antiprotrusio cage.

Christie MJ, Barrington SA, Brinson MF, Ruhling ME, DeBoer DK. Bridging massive acetabular defects with the triflange cup: 2- to 9-year results. Clin Orthop Relat Res. 2001;(393):216–27.

The triflange cup offers an alternative method of repair that reliably provides pain relief, initial implant stability, potential long-term implant stability, and pelvic stability in cases of discontinuity.

Gill TJ, Sledge JB, Müller ME: The Bürch-Schneider anti-protrusio cage in revision total hip arthroplasty. J Bone Joint Surg [Br]. 1998;80:946–53.

At an average follow-up of 8.5 years (5 to 18), 15 patients (25.9%) rated their results as excellent, 38 (65.5%) as good, and 5 (8.6%) as fair. Five further revisions of the acetabular prosthesis were required, three due to aseptic loosening, one for recurrent dislocation, and one due to sepsis. Of the remainder, 1 was definitely loose, 2 probably loose, and 12 possibly so. Impressive augmentation of bone stock can be achieved with the antiprotrusio cage, while enabling the hip to be centered in its anatomic position.

Gill TJ, Sledge JB, Müller ME: The management of severe acetabular bone loss using structural allograft and acetabular reinforcement devices. J Arthroplasty. 2000;15: 1–7.

This is the first reported series on the use of acetabular reinforcement devices with solid bulk allograft covering more than 50% of the socket. The allograft is protected in the early postoperative period, superior migration of the cup is virtually eliminated as a complication, and the incidence of aseptic loosening is greatly diminished.

Glassman AH, Engh CA, Bobyn JD. A technique of extensile exposure for total hip arthroplasty. J Arthroplasty. 1987;2:11–21.

The approach is based on the preservation of an intact musculo-osseous–muscular sleeve comprising the gluteus medius, greater trochanter, and vastus lateralis and allows physiologic reconstruction of the hip's soft tissue envelope. This versatile approach is particularly useful in revision surgery and in difficult primary interventions in which leg length is adjusted. The surgical technique, indications, and advantages are described. Early clinical results of 90 cases are presented.

Goodman S, Saastamoinen H, Shasha N, Gross AE. Complications of ilioischial reconstruction rings in revision total hip surgery. J Arthroplasty. 2004;19:436–46.

This paper recommends a constrained liner to avoid dislocation in selected cases, slotting the flange into the ischium for further stability, and protection of the sciatic nerve.

Korovessis P, Stamatakis M, Baikousis A, Katonis P, Petsinis G. Müller roof reinforcement rings: medium term results. Clin Orthop Relat Res. 1999;362:125–37.

In this small series, this surgical technique was successful and effective and followed by good medium-term clinical and radiographic results in primary and revision implantation in segmental, cavitary, or complex acetabular deficiencies and in osteoporotic or deficient acetabular bone.

Morsi E, Garbuz D, Gross AE. Revision total hip arthroplasty with shelf bulk allografts: a long term follow-up study. J Arthroplasty. 1996;11:86–90.

The use of bulk allograft in conjunction with acetabular revision is supported, provided that at least 50% support of the cup can be obtained with host bone. This type of reconstruction provides support for the cup and restores anatomy, leg length, and bone stock should future revision be necessary.

Perka C, Ludwig R. Reconstruction of segmental defects during revision procedures of the acetabulum with the Bürch-Schneider anti-protrusio cage. J Arthroplasty. 2001;16:568–74.

The cage has the lowest migration and loosening rate in cases with medial defects or anterior column defects. Surgical treatment of defects of the posterior column is associated with an increased rate of aseptic loosening, whereas implantation with cranial defects shows a higher migration rate with no significant increase in loosening.

Saleh KJ, Jaroszynski G, Woodgate I, Saleh L, Gross AE. Revision total hip arthroplasty with the use of structural acetabular allograft and reconstruction ring: a case series with a 10-year average follow-up. J Arthroplasty. 2000;15:951–8.

The study supports the use of massive structural allografts and reconstruction rings and achieved satisfactory results in 77% (10 of 13) of the patients. These results reveal an impressive outcome for what used to be thought of as a salvage operation.

Shinar AA, Harris WH. Bulk structural autogenous grafts and allografts for reconstruction of the acetabulum in total hip arthroplasty: sixteen-year average follow-up. J Bone Joint Surg [Am]. 1997;79:159–68.

Both the structural autogenous grafts and the structural allografts used in acetabular reconstruction in total hip replacement functioned well for the initial 5–10 years. At an average of 16.5 years, 9 of the 15 hips treated with allograft and 16 (29%) of the 55 treated with autogenous graft had been revised. The greater the extent of coverage of the acetabular component by the graft, the greater the rate of late failure.

Winter E, Piert M, Volkmann R, Maurer F, Eingartner C, Weise K, Weller S. Allogeneic cancellous bone graft and a Bürch-Schneider ring for acetabular reconstruction in revision hip arthroplasty. J Bone Joint Surg [Am]. 2001;83:862–7.

Acetabular reconstruction with the use of morselized cryopreserved allogeneic cancellous bone graft and the Bürch-Schneider ring can be highly successful in managing massive acetabular deficiencies in revision hip arthroplasty.

Woodgate IG, Saleh KJ, Jaroszynski G, Agnidis Z, Woodgate MM, Gross AE. Minor column structural acetabular allografts in revision hip arthroplasty. Clin Orthop Relat Res. 2000;371:75–85.

The study shows that good results can be achieved with structural acetabular allograft reconstruction supporting less than 50% of the cup, with good mid-term to long-term implant survival (cup aseptic survival, 80.4%; allograft reconstruction survival, 94.1%), especially if there is restoration of near-normal hip biomechanics.

Zehntner MK, Ganz R. Midterm results (5.5–10 years) of acetabular allograft reconstruction with the acetabular reinforcement ring during total hip revision. J Arthroplasty. 1994;9:469–79.

Kaplan-Meier survivorship analysis revealed a 79.6% probability of reconstruction survival at 10 years with revision as the end point for failure. It was concluded that durability of the reconstruction can be expected if support of the metallic reinforcement device is provided by host bone. Segmental and combined deficiencies may require additional internal fixation by plates and screws.

Femoral Revision: Impaction Grafting

John A. F. Charity, A. John Timperley, and Graham A. Gie

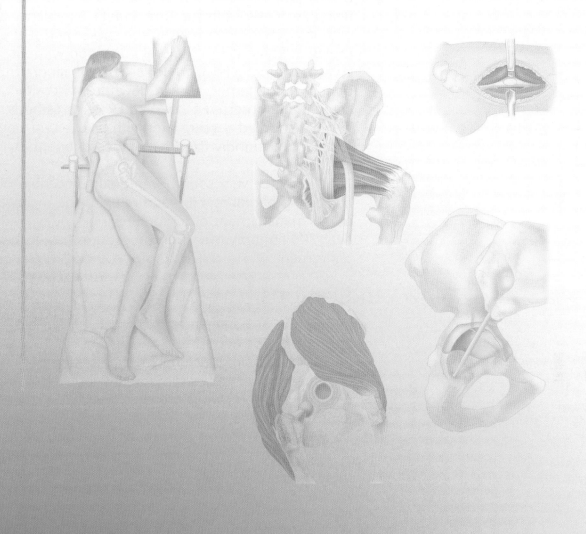

Introduction

- Femoral impaction bone grafting in revision hip surgery, accompanied by cementing of a femoral stem, was first introduced into clinical practice in Exeter in April 1987.
- Graham Gie, while on a 1-year hip fellowship, was faced with a second revision hip replacement in an elderly lady in whom femoral bone stock was poor. Being aware of Professor Tom Slooff's experience with impaction bone graft in the socket and Professor Robin Ling's femoral impaction without cement, he proceeded to impact milled allograft bone into the femur, sucked down low-viscosity cement, and inserted a polished Exeter prosthesis. The patient died 5 years later with recovery of bone stock and a soundly fixed femoral component in position.
- The technique very soon became our procedure of choice in femoral revision and remains the mainstay of our management of femoral revision today, with over 700 femoral impaction procedures having been performed.

Indications

- Restoration of bone stock in femoral revision hip arthroplasty
- Provision of an interface for mechanical interlocking of cement in cemented femoral revision where removal of the previous prosthesis has left a smooth endosteal surface
- To avoid the insertion of distal fixation long stems in young patients in whom later further revision surgery might be compromised
- Where the required length of "scratch fit" cannot be achieved with a fully coated cementless stem
- Where the intramedullary canal diameter is greater than 18 mm, in which situation it is known that uncemented stems have a high incidence of thigh pain
- Where fixation with a coned fluted stem cannot be achieved due to the reverse cone shape of the natural femur below the isthmus

PITFALLS

- *In cases in which complete loss of the proximal femur exceeds 10 cm*

- *Very elderly patients in whom bone stock recovery is not an issue*

- *Medically unfit patients in whom a relatively short revision operation is desirable*

Controversies

- Age limit and life expectancy; physiologic age rather than chronologic age should be considered.

Examination/Imaging

- Anteroposterior pelvis radiographs for hips
  - Anteroposterior hip radiograph to include the tip of the prosthesis and to beyond distal cement if present. This radiograph allows one to determine instruments required for prosthesis removal (e.g., long drills, ultrasound cement removal instruments) and whether extended trochanteric osteotomy will be required for implant removal. In Figure 1A, lysis does not extend beyond the distal half of the stem, so a standard length stem can be used in this revision.
  - Lateral hip radiograph to include the tip of the stem and show its relationship to the inner femoral cortex (Fig. 1B). This radiograph allows one to assess risk of femoral penetration during implant and particularly cement removal. The tip of the stem in Figure 1 is in the center of the canal, so the surgeon can confidently drill the distal cement mantle without fear of cortical penetration.
  - Radiographs also allow one to assess the need for prophylactic diaphyseal femoral wiring, meshing of diaphyseal defects, and proximal femoral reconstruction (e.g., calcar deficiency as in Fig. 1).
- Exclusion of infection by appropriate blood tests, hip aspiration, and isotope scanning

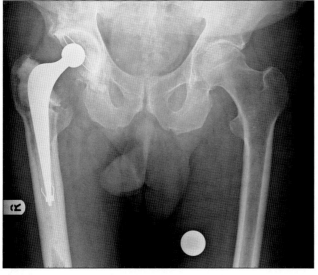
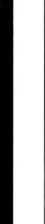

A
B

FIGURE 1

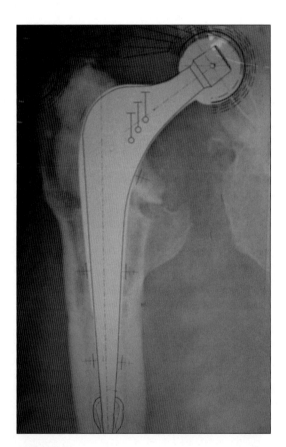

Treatment Options

- Depending on patient's age, general health, bone quality, and extent of bone lysis, other treatment options include:
  - Cemented femoral stem, short or long
  - Cementless femoral stem (of multiple designs and coatings)
  - Proximal femoral replacement
  - Tumor prosthesis

TEMPLATING (Fig. 2)

- To assess leg length discrepancy, required femoral component size, offset, and length and to ensure chosen length bypasses bone lysis areas by at least two cortical diameters or, if this is not possible, to ensure the availability of cortical struts to reinforce the weakened bone areas
- To determine depth within the femur to which threaded revision plug needs to be placed

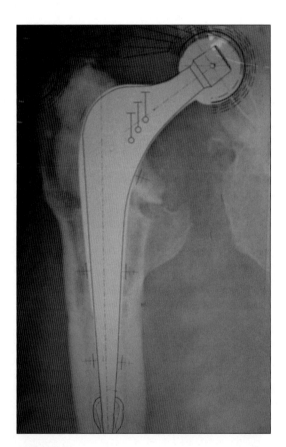

FIGURE 2

Surgical Anatomy

- Ensure identification and exposure of the sciatic nerve (posterior approach).
- Avoid a proximal split in the gluteus medius muscle to prevent damage to the superior gluteal nerve and artery (lateral approach).
- Cut the external rotator muscles as close to their femoral insertion as possible and perform detailed repair on closure (posterior approach).
- Perform careful bony repair of the gluteus medius and minimus tendons (lateral approach).

Positioning

- The lateral position is routinely used.
- Supports are placed on both anterior superior iliac spines (ASISs) and posteriorly on the sacrum for firm fixation (Fig. 3A and 3B).
  - Care should be taken to avoid excessive pressure on the ASIS as postoperative troublesome meralgia paresthetica can result.
  - Sacral support should be placed fairly low in case incision needs to be extended into the buttock for acetabular reconstruction.

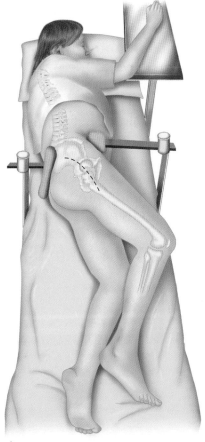

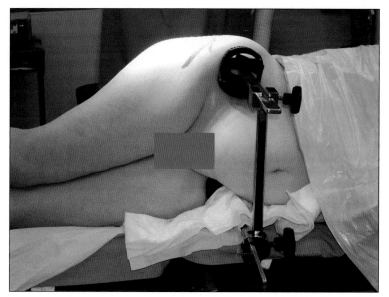

A　　　　　　　B

FIGURE 3

Portals/Exposures

- In our institution, the posterior approach is routinely used for revision hip surgery.
- There is no place for minimal incision surgery or minimally invasive surgery in femoral revision with impaction grafting.
- The surgical assistant must be able to hold the limb in the required position without any torque on the femoral shaft; otherwise, a spiral fracture will occur during forceful impaction. Release of all the external hip rotators, psoas tendon, gluteus maximus insertion into the femur, and anterior capsule is usually required to achieve this.
- Draping should ensure that exposure to the supracondylar area is possible should that become necessary during the procedure.

Procedure

STEP 1: INSERTION OF THREADED PLUG

- In femoral impaction bone grafting, the bone chips need to be in contact with host bone over the largest possible surface area, and therefore all debris and old cement needs to be removed from the femoral canal. The only exception to this is cement that lies two cortical diameters beyond the most distal lytic area in the femur. In the absence of infection, this cement can be safely left.
- During final debris removal, femoral canal reamers are used. The largest reamer used will determine the size of femoral plug required.
- The appropriately sized femoral impaction plug (Fig. 4A) is fixed to a threaded guidewire and inserted to the templated depth using the revision plug introducer (Fig. 4B), which is then removed (Fig. 5A), leaving the guidewire in place (Fig. 5B).

PEARLS

- *If the plug attached to the guidewire with depth markers is inserted to a depth that takes it beyond the isthmus, it will not fix firmly in the canal. A second guidewire is then placed externally along the femur to the same depth and the plug is then skewered percutaneously with a 2-mm Kirschner wire. This wire is left protruding from the skin for removal at the end of the procedure.*

- *If there is well-fixed cement lying two cortical diameters beyond the distal-most lytic lesion in the femur, it can be used as a plug for the graft by drilling it centrally using a long drill through the largest distal femoral impactor that will fit into the femur and onto the cement. The threaded guidewire can then be screwed directly into the cement.*

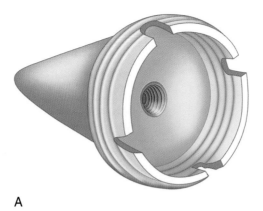

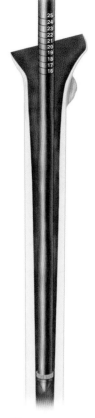

FIGURE 4

B

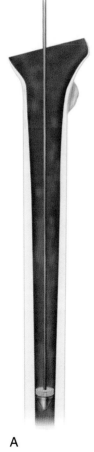

A

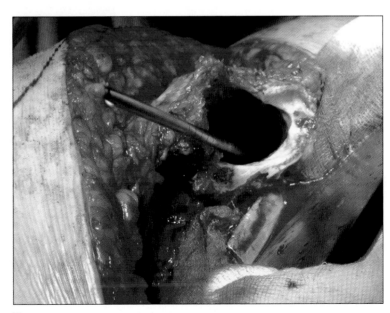

B

FIGURE 5

STEP 2: SIZING THE FEMORAL CANAL

- The proximal femoral impactor ("phantom") of the templated size and offset is passed over the guide rod to ensure that it will seat easily to the required level (Fig. 6A and 6B). If there is any bony obstruction to its passage, then a smaller size should be selected.

- Before using the distal impactors to impact the bone chips, it is important to establish the distance down the canal that each size of impactor can be passed without jamming in the canal and potentially causing a fracture. Select a distal impactor one size smaller in diameter than the intramedullary plug diameter. This should pass easily over the guidewire down to the plug without obstruction. Withdraw this impactor 2 cm and snap on a plastic marker clip at the level of the greater trochanter to mark the intended depth of insertion. This will create a 2-cm distal bone plug and reduce the risk of the canal plug being driven further down the femur.

- Larger diameter impactors are in turn introduced as far down the canal as they will pass and similarly marked with a clip (Fig. 7A and 7B). When subsequently impacting the bone chips, do not drive the impactors beyond this marked depth.

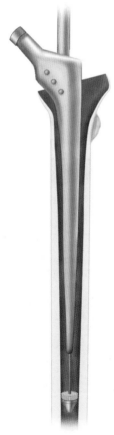

A

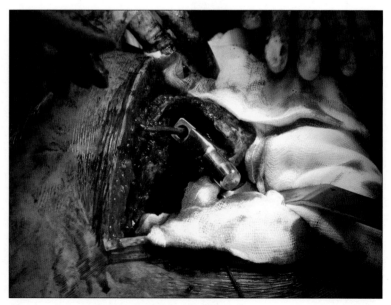

B

FIGURE 6

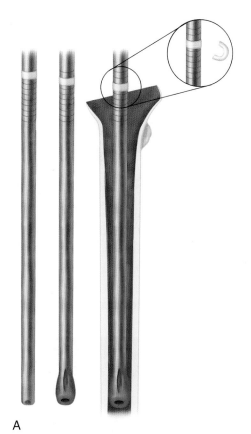

A

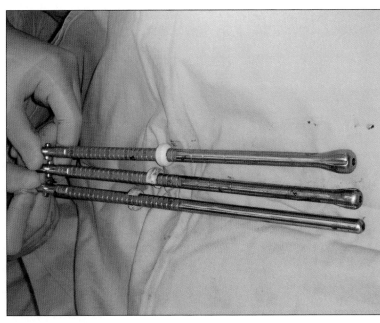

B

FIGURE 7

STEP 3: DISTAL IMPACTION

- Two-millimeter to 4-mm cancellous bone chips are introduced into the canal using an open-ended syringe (Fig. 8).
- Prior to commencement of bone impaction, diaphyseal defects must be repaired. Appropriate wire meshes are used (Fig. 9).
- Chips are driven distally using the distal impactors to the depth of the plastic markers (Fig. 10). Progressively larger impactors are used as the canal is filled.
- More chips are introduced and impacted extremely firmly until the impactors cannot be driven beyond the distal impaction line (junction of polished and ridged sections of impactor) (Fig. 11). Impaction with the phantoms is then commenced.

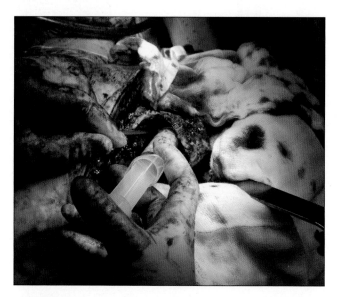

FIGURE 8

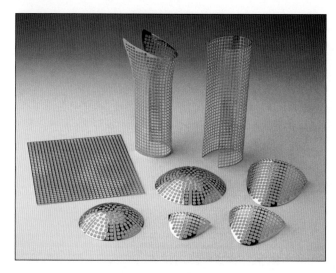

FIGURE 9

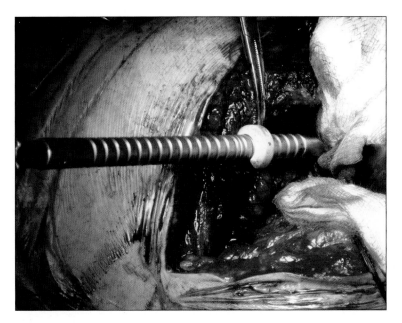

FIGURE 10

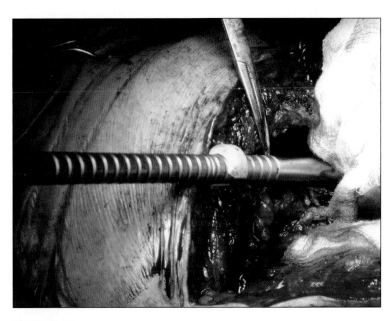

FIGURE 11

STEP 4: IMPACTION USING THE PHANTOMS

- The phantom, which is exactly the same shape as the final prosthesis but oversized to allow for an adequate cement mantle, is then hammered into the distally impacted bone and then removed.
- Further graft is added, driven into the diaphysis with hand-held distal impactors, and the phantom reinserted. The procedure is repeated until the phantom is stable enough to perform a trial reduction, when stability and leg length can be assessed. The relationship of the phantom to host bone is marked with methylene blue dye for later reference.
- The requirement for calcar reconstruction can be reassessed at this time and is strongly recommended if there is less than 1 cm of medial femoral neck above the lesser trochanter and if the cortical bone does not at least reach the most distal leg length mark on the prosthesis. The appropriately shaped metal mesh is wired in position (Fig. 12A and 12B).
- The impaction process is then repeated until graft is firmly impacted to within 1–2 cm of the top of the calcar/wire mesh (Fig. 13). At this stage it should be impossible to withdraw the phantom by hand; it should only be removable using the slap-hammer.

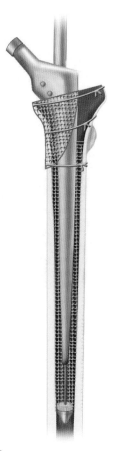

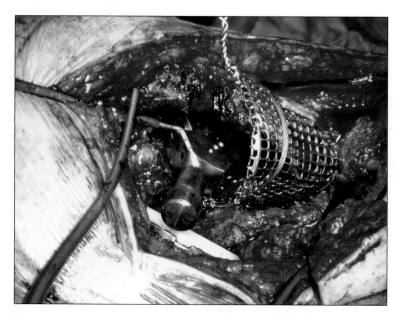

A   B

FIGURE 12

- *If at trial reduction the leg is found to be too long or the reduction too tight, and the phantom is so tight it cannot be hammered any deeper, then it should be removed and a phantom one size smaller inserted. The surgeon then has the option of using the smaller prosthesis or hammering it deeper than required and reinserting the larger component.*

- *Test that the phantom is not removable by hand. If it is, further impaction is required.*

- *Do not apply the calcar mesh before trial reduction as this may lead to insufficient build-up of the calcar or excessive build-up such that the metal mesh comes into contact with the prosthesis. Calcar reconstruction is only performed once final position of the prosthesis has been determined.*

- *Apply the calcar mesh with the phantom in position as this will avoid overtightening and resultant contact between mesh and prosthesis.*

- *Check that the methylene blue dye mark is still visible, as it is often covered by proximal reconstruction. If not, repeat the trial reduction and re-mark.*

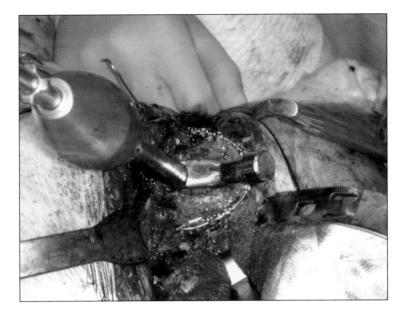

FIGURE 13

- *If the distal canal is overfilled (i.e., to above the level of the distal impaction line), then it will be impossible to insert the phantom to the required depth.*

- *Failure to recognize a calcar or diaphyseal fracture. If ever the phantom is felt to insert easier than it did with the previous impaction, a fracture is present and must be identified and wired.*

- *Failure to build up calcar sufficiently, resulting in inadequate femoral component rotational stability.*

- *If the phantom is removable by hand, impaction is inadequate.*

STEP 5: PROXIMAL IMPACTION

- This step is probably the most important part of the procedure, allowing for the transmission of load into the upper end of the femur and ensuring that prosthesis subsidence is no more than one would expect to see in primary hip surgery.
- Using the proximal impactors and large cancellous chips (8–10 mm in diameter), hammer the chips firmly around the phantom until level with the top of the host bone/calcar mesh (Fig. 14A and 14B). At this stage the phantom should be absolutely rotationally stable within the femur and the impacted bone.
- Back the phantom out 2 cm, apply more large chips, hammer the chips firmly, and then drive the phantom back in to the correct depth (Fig. 15A and 15B).
- Calcar mesh wires are further tightened.

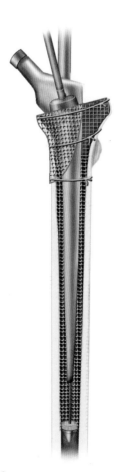

A

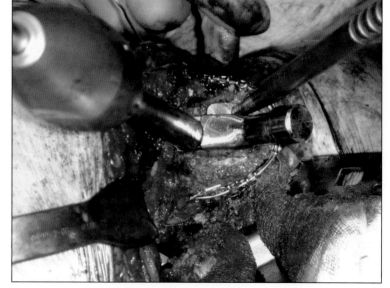

B

FIGURE 14

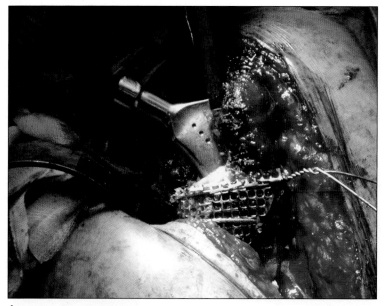

A

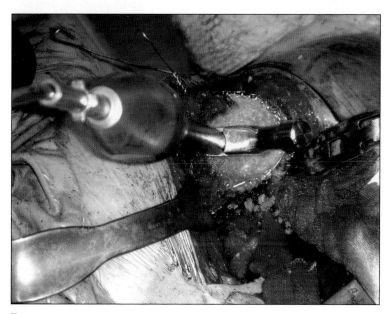

B

FIGURE 15

STEP 6: CEMENTING AND STEM INSERTION

- The threaded guidewire is unscrewed from the plug and removed.
- A suction catheter is inserted down the phantom to suck the canal dry distally (Fig. 16).
- Cement is mixed in a cement gun with a narrow or tapered spout.
- The phantom is removed immediately prior to cement injection and the suction catheter reinserted. Note the neomedullary canal in Figure 17.
- Cement is injected retrograde, removing the suction catheter as soon as it blocks.

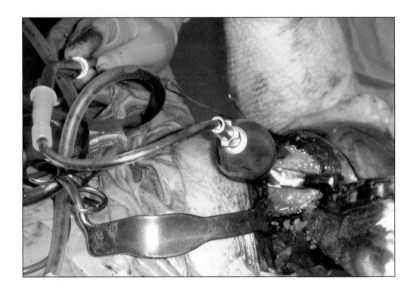

FIGURE 16

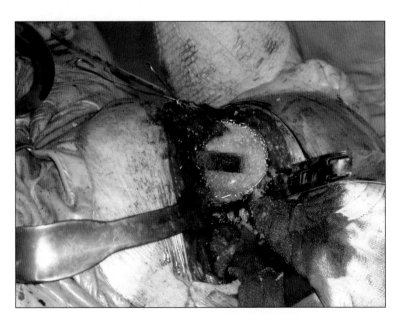

FIGURE 17

- A proximal femoral seal is applied to the gun spout and the spout cut short.
- Cement is firmly pressurized (Fig. 18A) and the definitive stem inserted to the predetermined and marked depth as the viscosity of the cement starts increasing (Fig. 18B).

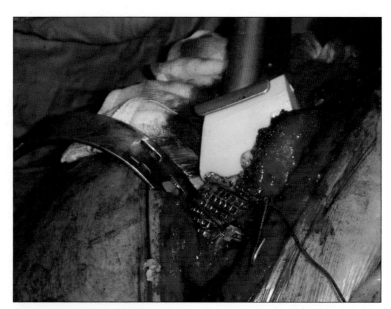

A

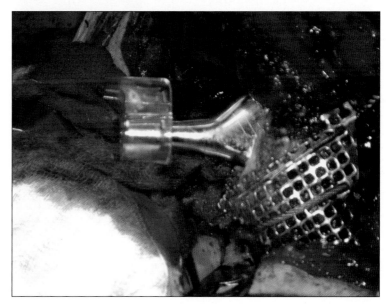

B

FIGURE 18

- The introducer is removed and a "horse collar" applied (Fig. 19A) until the cement has cured (Fig. 19B).
- Final tightening of the calcar wires is done.
- The appropriate femoral head is applied, the hip is reduced, and the external rotators are repaired; wound closure is done by the surgeon's preferred method. The postoperative results can be reviewed on anteroposterior (Fig. 20A) and lateral (Fig. 20B) radiographs.
- Drains are no longer routinely used, and their requirement is assessed on a per case basis.

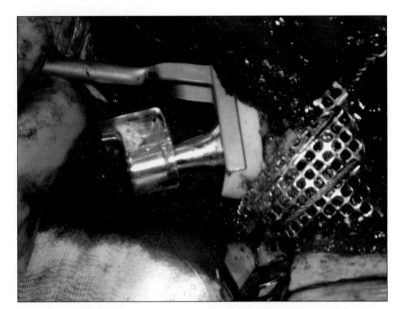

A

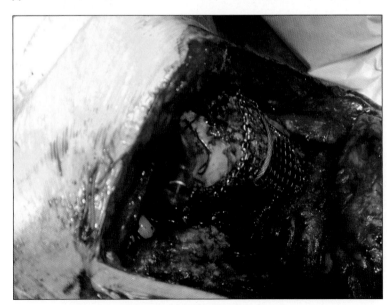

B

FIGURE 19

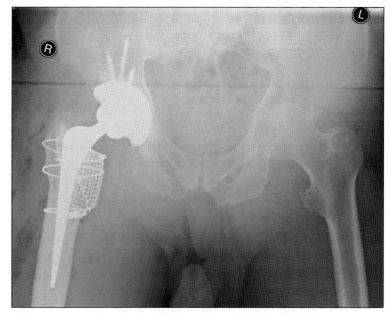

A

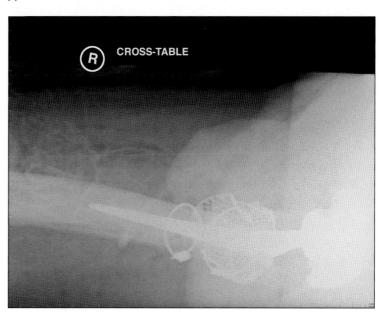

CROSS-TABLE

B

FIGURE 20

Complications

- Potential complications are as for revision hip surgery in general, including dislocation (most common complication), femoral fracture, deep venous thrombosis, pulmonary embolus, sepsis, nerve palsies, and mortality.

Postoperative Care and Expected Outcomes

- In our institute, revision hip surgery is usually carried out under epidural and light general anesthesia. Mobilization is commenced after removal of the epidural cannula, usually at 48 hours.
- The degree of weight bearing is usually governed by the procedure carried out on the acetabular side.
  - With reasonable bone stock, full weight bearing is permitted immediately as comfortable.
  - If bone stock is particularly flimsy, crutches and restricted weight bearing are encouraged for 6–12 weeks.
- In our experience, the procedure is well tolerated with little early postoperative discomfort.
- At 15 years, survivorship of the stem with re-operation of the femoral side for any reason as the end point is 82% and survivorship with aseptic loosening of the stem as the end point is 98.5%.

Evidence

Bolder SB, Schreurs BW, Verdonschot N, Veth RP, Buma P. Wire mesh allows more revascularisation than a strut in impaction bone grafting: an animal study in goats. Clin Orthop Relat Res. 2004;(423):280–6.

Medial femoral neck defects were created in goat femora. These were then reconstructed with wire mesh or with strut grafts prior to impaction grafting. Deep to the strut grafts, no revascularization was seen at 6 weeks. In the mesh group, fibrous tissue and blood vessels penetrated the mesh and a superficial zone of revascularized grafts was observed.

English H, Timperley A, Dunlop D, Gie G. Impaction grafting of the femur in two-stage revision for infected total hip replacement. J Bone Joint Surg [Br]. 2002;84:809–17.

This paper reports the results of 53 Femoral Impaction Grafts (FIG) done at the second stage of a two-stage revision for infection. It demonstrates that it is safe to perform FIG following infected THR with a success rate of 93% in the elimination of infection at a mean follow-up of 53 months.

Gie GA, Linder L, Ling RS, Simon JP, Slooff TJ, Timperley AJ. Impacted cancellous allograft and cement for revision total hip arthroplasty. J Bone Joint Surg [Br]. 1993;75:14–21.

This is the first detailed publication of the results of femoral impaction grafting. The first 68 cases operated on for femoral component loosening are reported with 56 cases being reviewed with a follow-up of 18 to 49 months. Relief of symptoms and functional results were found to compare well with those of primary arthroplasty, with a low complication rate and evidence of graft healing.

Giesen EB, Lamerigts NM, Verdonschot N, Buma P, Schreurs BW, Huiskes R. Mechanical characteristics of impacted morsellised bone grafts used in revision of total hip arthroplasty. J Bone Joint Surg [Br]. 1999;81:1052–7.

The aim of this study was to document the time-dependent mechanical properties of morcellized bone graft. The authors concluded that in clinical use the graft is bound to be subject to permanent deformation after operation. The confined compression modulus was found to be low relative to cancellous bone. Designs of prostheses used with impaction grafting must therefore accommodate the viscoelastic and permanent deformations in the graft without causing loosening at the interface.

Halliday BR, English HW, Timperley AJ, Gie GA, Ling RS. Femoral impaction grafting with cement in revision total hip replacement: evolution of the technique and results. J Bone Joint Surg [Br]. 2003;85:809–17.

The results of femoral impaction grafting with a minimum follow-up of 5 years are reported. Two hundred twenty-six hips in 207 patients were studied. At 10 to 11 years, survivorship with reoperation for femoral loosening as the endpoint was 99.1% and that for any femoral reoperation, 90.5%. The incidence of postoperative femoral shaft fractures encouraged the use of longer stems.

Ling RS, Timperley AJ, Linder L. Histology of cancellous impaction grafting in the femur: a case report. J Bone Joint Surg [Br]. 1993;75:693–6.

This post-mortem study reports on the histology of a femur retrieved 3.5 years after impaction femoral bone grafting. Two large femoral defects had been covered with wire mesh to contain the impacted bone. The macroscopic specimen showed that cortical bone had reformed and histology showed that the allograft chips had been replaced by viable cortical bone.

Schreurs BW, Arts C, Verdonschot N, Buma P, Slooff TJ, Gardeniers JW. Femoral component revision with use of impaction bone-grafting and a cemented polished stem. J Bone Joint Surg [Am]. 2005;87:2499–507.

Thirty-three consecutive femoral impaction grafts using a cemented polished Exeter stem were reviewed 8 to 13 years postoperatively. No femoral reconstruction had been re-revised for any reason at a mean of 10.4 years.

Ullmark G, Nilsson O. Impacted corticocancellous allografts: recoil and strength. J Arthroplasty. 1999;14:1019–23.

For this in-vitro study, bone grafts were morcellized to produce chips of two different ranges of sizes. These were impacted with two different impaction forces. There was less subsidence with the bigger type of bone chips and with the harder impacted graft beds.

ACKNOWLEDGMENTS

The authors would like to thank Mrs. Paula Charity for producing the original illustrations, Mrs. Sophie Kolowska for taking the photographs, and the Exeter Hip Foundation for releasing the illustrations and photographs for publication.

Femoral Stem Revision: Posterior Approach

Oliver Keast-Butler and James P. Waddell

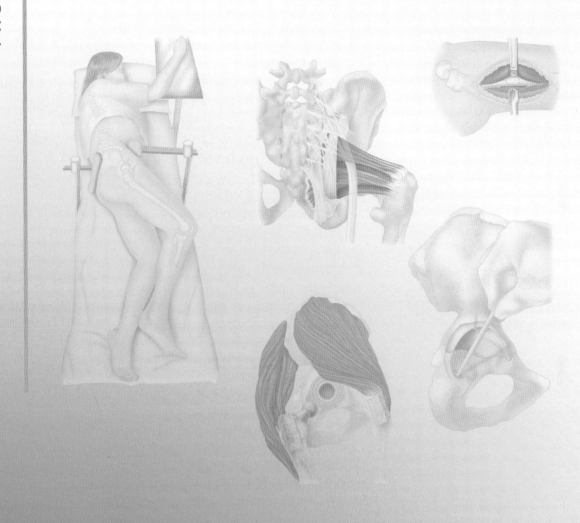

Controversies

- We prefer the posterior approach, irrespective of the previous approach(s).
  - In revision of a previous lateral approach, it avoids further damage to the gluteus medius and minimus, which have often not healed (see Fig. 2).
  - It allows extensile exposure of the acetabulum. The excellent femoral exposure often allows implant removal without the need for femoral/trochanteric osteotomy and its related morbidity.
  - In revising failed internal fixation of hip fractures, the approach can be performed and the hip dislocated prior to removal of metalwork, which requires minimal further dissection.

Treatment Options

- Lateral approach
- Anterolateral approach

Indications

- Revision of failed primary hip replacement
- Second-stage revision of infected hip replacement
- Revision of failed proximal femoral fracture fixation

Examination/Imaging

- Anteroposterior and lateral radiographs of the pelvis and femur
- Preoperative templating and planning
  - Is the stem to be revised cemented or uncemented?
  - Is the stem or cement loose? If the stem or cement is loose, it can be removed straightforwardly.
  - Has a varus femoral deformity occurred?
  - If distal cement and/or a sclerotic bone pedestal is present, it can be removed with the aid of a bone window.
  - If removing a well-fixed stem, an extended trochanteric osteotomy may be required.
  - Ensure familiarity with the revision system.
  - Ensure that inventory allows for revision of all components with compatible head sizes if the acetabulum is to be retained.
  - Be prepared for intraoperative complications such as fracture.

Surgical Anatomy

- See posterior approach for primary hip replacement in Procedure 5.
- To increase exposure, the quadratus femoris and gluteus major insertion into gluteal tuberosity on the femur can be divided, leaving residual soft tissue stumps attached to the femur for repair.
- If an extended trochanteric osteotomy or distal window is required, the vastus lateralis can be elevated from the intramuscular septum, allowing extensile exposure of the femur from the hip to the knee.
- We do not routinely expose the sciatic nerve, releasing scar tissue and pseudo-capsule from the posterior intertrochanteric line and reflecting this flap posteriorly as one layer with the nerve remaining behind it.

Positioning

- The patient is placed in the lateral decubitus position.
- The pelvis is secured with anterior and posterior bolsters resting on the pubis and sacrum.
- The trunk is secured with anterior and posterior bolsters at the sternum and scapulae.
- An axillary bump is used to decrease pressure on the inferior arm.
- Prep and drape the lower limb allowing access to the entire femur.

Portals/Exposures

- Make the skin incision, a longitudinal incision with a posterior curve proximally toward the posterior superior iliac spine.
  - Center the incision over the posterior third of the greater trochanter. Use the old scar if it is in a reasonable position.
  - If revising a previous lateral approach, the surgeon may need to use a new incision or modify the old one (Fig. 1).

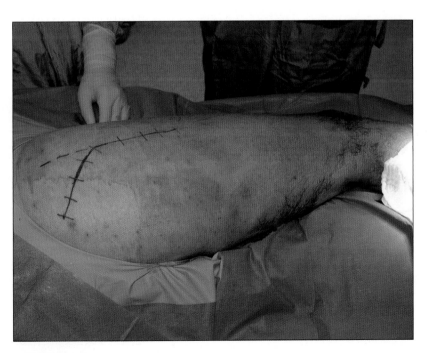

FIGURE 1

- Expose the fascia lata or gluteus maximus fascia, which may be significantly scarred.
  - Do not create skin flaps or undermine the incision.
  - Incise the fascia or split the gluteus maximus in the line of the skin incision (Fig. 2).
  - Blunt dissection with a finger underneath the fascia will expose the vastus lateralis and gluteus medius, which are often adherent to the fascia lata.
- Internally rotate the femur to put posterior tissue under tension.
- Place a retractor deep to the gluteus medius and gently retract the muscle (Fig. 3).
- If revising a previous lateral approach, with anatomy similar to that in a primary hip replacement (see Fig. 3), the posterior capsule is seen after division of the short rotators (Fig. 4).
- If revising a previous posterior approach, the piriformis and short rotators may not be evident. In this case, divide short rotators and capsule from the femoral insertion as one layer, proximally from the free edge of the gluteus medius distally to the quadratus femoris or gluteus maximus tendon if the former muscle is poorly defined scar tissue.
- The sciatic nerve is less apparent than in primary hip replacement and is palpated but not explored.
- After incising the posterior capsule, with internal rotation to maintain tissue tension, the femoral head and acetabular component will come into view. Preserve the posterior tissue for later repair.

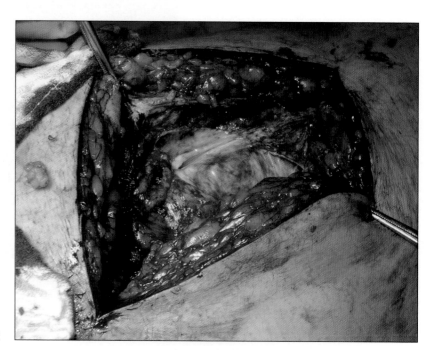

FIGURE 2

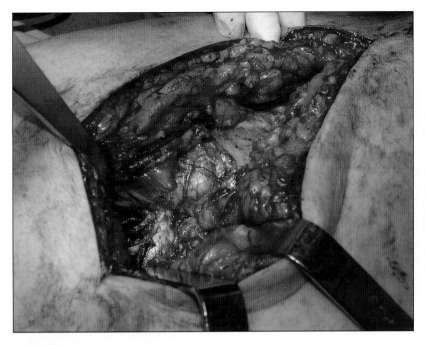

FIGURE 3

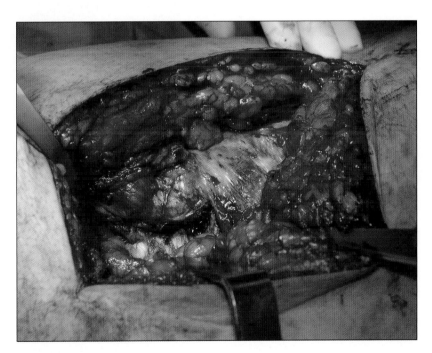

FIGURE 4

- Place retractors anterosuperiorly over the superior acetabulum, and inferiorly over the posterior column of the acetabulum. Excise inferior and anterior scar tissue and/or capsule and place a further retractor anterior to the anterior acetabular wall.
- Once the acetabulum is exposed, posterior dislocation of the hip is usually straightforward (Fig. 5).
- Remove the modular femoral head if present and confirm head size.
- Retractors placed around the inferior femoral neck allow the neck to be dissected free.
- Dissect soft tissue from the bone-prosthesis interfaces of the femur and acetabulum to assess bone loss and implant stability.

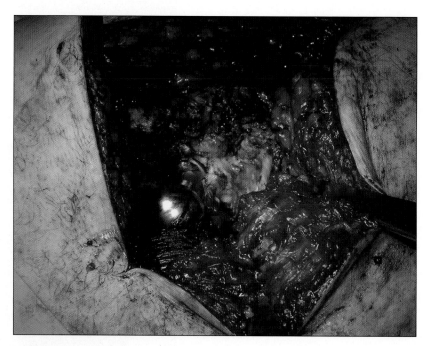

FIGURE 5

Procedure

STEP 1: REMOVAL OF FEMORAL STEM

- Dislocate the hip and remove the modular head.
- Excise tissue at the bone-prosthesis interface.
- Remove bone and/or cement from the shoulders of the prosthesis.
- Remove proximal cement (if revising a cemented prosthesis).
- Use flexible osteotomes to cut the proximal bone-prosthesis interface.

- A cemented or loose uncemented stem can then be removed with an extraction device with force directed along the line of the intramedullary canal (Fig. 6).
- If the stem can't be removed, consider an extended trochanteric osteotomy.

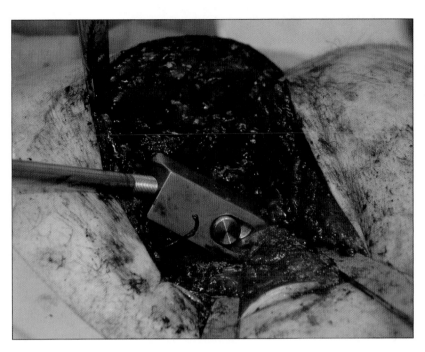

FIGURE 6

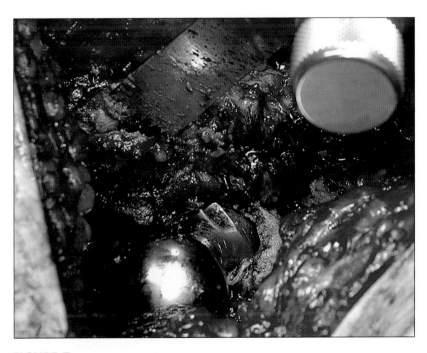

FIGURE 7

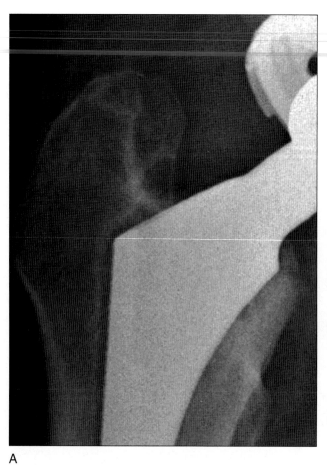
A

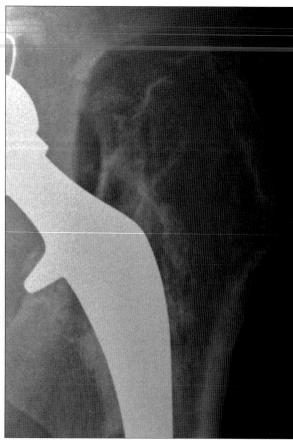
B

FIGURE 8

PITFALLS

• *Incomplete removal of proximal bone and/or cement may result in a trochanteric fracture occurring during component removal (Fig. 9A and 9B).*

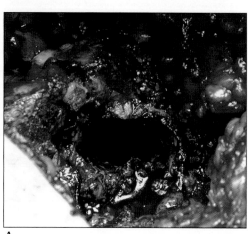

FIGURE 9   A   B

STEP 2: REMOVAL OF CEMENT RESTRICTOR/ DISTAL BONE PEDESTAL WITH BONE WINDOW

- In certain circumstances we use a cortical window on the lateral femoral cortex.
  - A cement restrictor and adjacent cement are often well fixed, even if proximal cement is loose (Fig. 10A and 10B).
  - In uncemented stem revision, a sclerotic pedestal may have formed at the tip of the prosthesis. This can make finding the distal canal difficult.

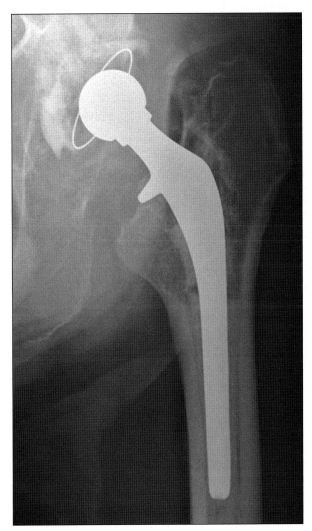

A

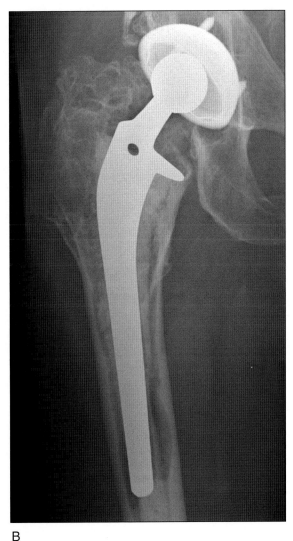

B

FIGURE 10

- • If the prosthesis tip is close to the anterior femoral cortex (Fig. 11), anterior cortical perforation may occur when drilling into the distal canal.
- The window should be at the junction of the cement restrictor and the distal canal. (Its distance from the greater trochanter should be determined during preoperative planning.)
- Elevate the vastus lateralis at the chosen level.
- Use a high-speed burr to cut an oval window 10–20 mm long×10 mm wide (less than one-third the circumference of the femur); remove the bone fragment and set aside.
- Small fragments of cement and restrictor are removed through the window.
- The window can facilitate drilling down the femoral canal and through the obstruction. At this point you can see that the drill is inside the distal femur.
- Bone and cement can be removed with hooks and cement removal instruments as preferred (Fig. 12).
- Prophylactic cerclage wire is placed distal to the window prior to stem insertion.
- Trials and the definitive stem are inserted under direct vision through the window (with >5 cm stem fixation distal to the window).

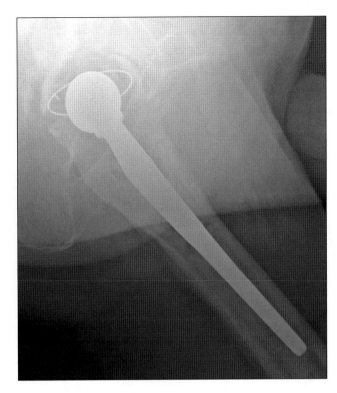

FIGURE 11

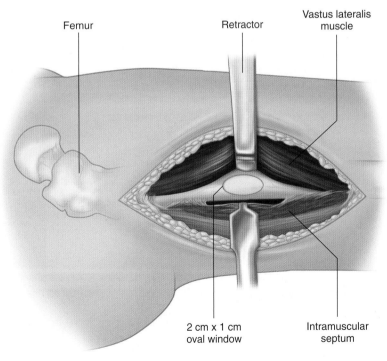

Femur   Retractor   Vastus lateralis
muscle

2 cm x 1 cm
oval window   Intramuscular
septum

FIGURE 12

- Resected bone window and graft obtained during femoral preparation can be replaced and held with cerclage wire (Fig. 13).
- A reinforcing strut allograft can be used if distal stem fixation is unsatisfactory (Fig. 14).

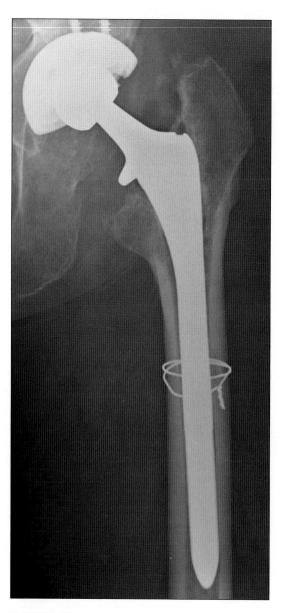

FIGURE 13

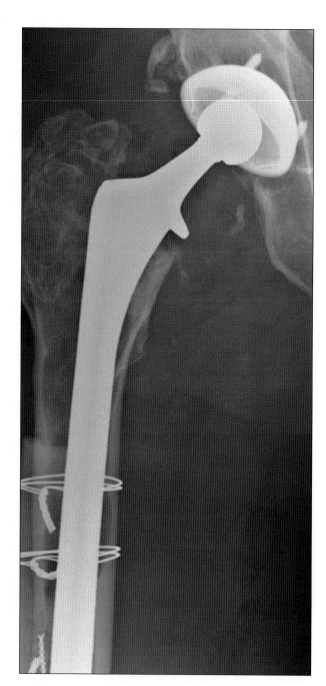

FIGURE 14

STEP 3: EXTENDED TROCHANTERIC OSTEOTOMY TO REMOVE WELL-FIXED STEM

- The length of the osteotomy is determined from preoperative templates.
- A standard posterior approach is used. Distal wound extension is made to the extent of the planned osteotomy (Fig. 15).

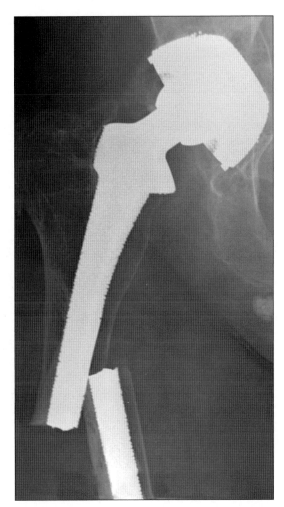

FIGURE 15

- Divide the gluteus maximus tendon midsubstance and elevate the vastus lateralis from the intramuscular septum, leaving a small cuff of muscle (Fig. 16).
- Use a saw or burr to release the lateral femoral cortex and greater trochanter (one third the diameter of the femoral shaft).
- Distally, curve the osteotomy to minimize risk of fracture propagation.
- Use osteotomes to carefully displace osteotomized bone (Fig. 17A and 17B).

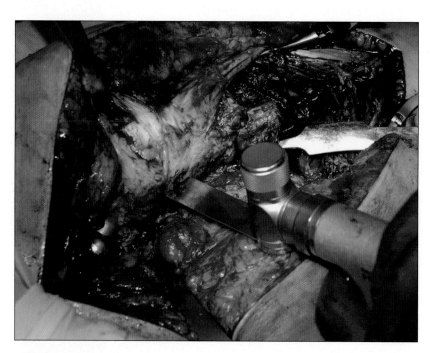

FIGURE 16

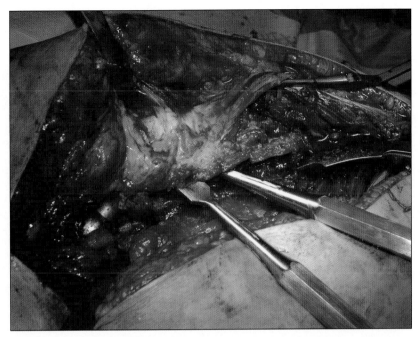

A

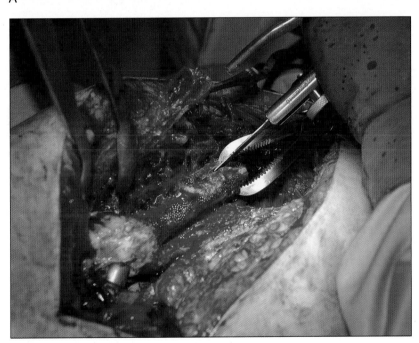

B

FIGURE 17

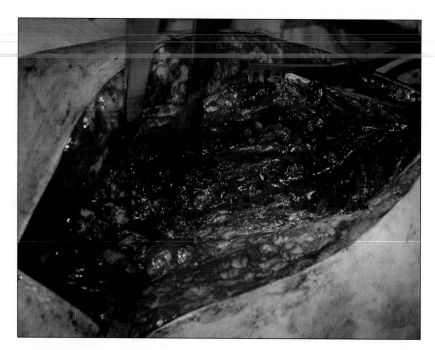

FIGURE 18

- Despite care, existing osteoporosis often results in a fragile residual shell after implant removal (Fig. 18).
- Removal of cylindrical sections of the prosthesis is done with thin curved osteotomes (Fig. 19A) and trephine drills (Fig. 19B).

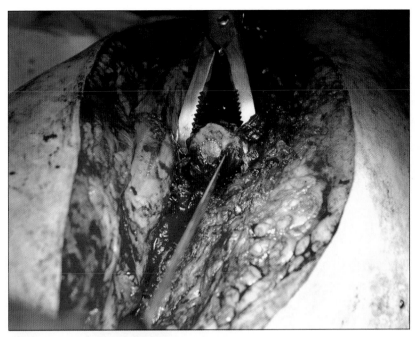

A

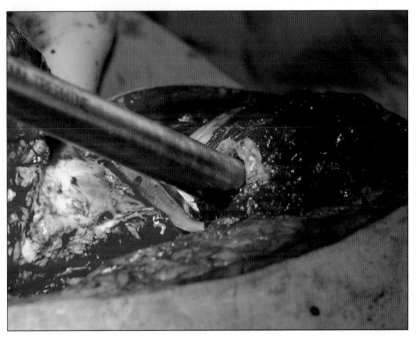

B

FIGURE 19

- Once advanced beyond the prosthesis tip, the drill pitch changes and the prosthesis usually comes out with removal of the trephine (Fig. 20).
- Following insertion of the definitive stem, the osteotomy is closed using cerclage wires (Fig. 21).
- Strut allograft can be used to restore bone stock and ensure that the stem is covered (Fig. 22). If allograft is used for mechanical strength, we use cables to fix it to the femur (Fig. 23A–23C).

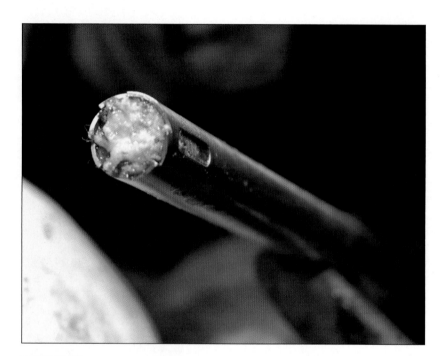

FIGURE 20

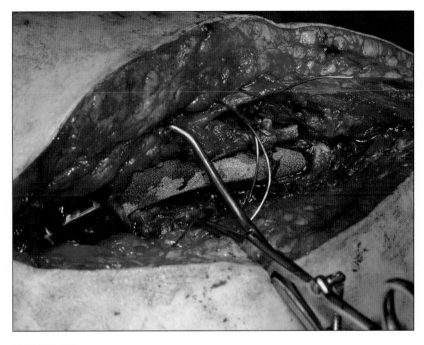

FIGURE 21

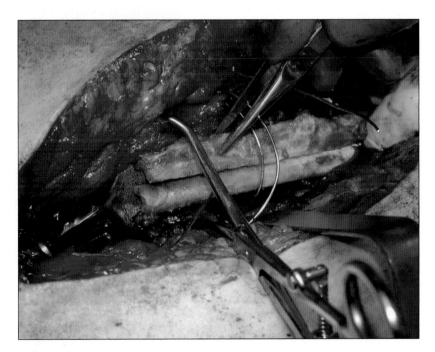

FIGURE 22

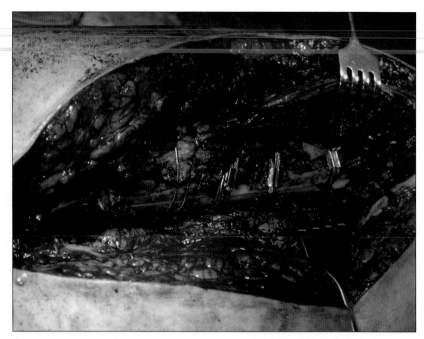

A

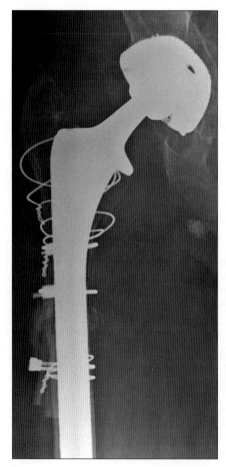

B   C

FIGURE 23

Step 4: Insertion of Definitive Component

- We prefer an extensively coated monoblock stem with distal flutes to improve rotational stability. This stem design is initially reliant on distal fixation and bypasses the abnormal bone.
- Stems greater than 190 mm are usually curved to prevent perforation of the anterior cortex. They require flexible reamers or narrow-stem reamers (Fig. 24) to negotiate the anterior femoral bow.
- We plan for 5 cm of diaphyseal press-fit beyond the femoral defect.
- Using straight hand reamers, ream sequentially to the desired size (usually 1–1.5 mm less than the final stem diameter). If good cortical "chatter" is not encountered, increase the diameter of the reamer and subsequent stem.

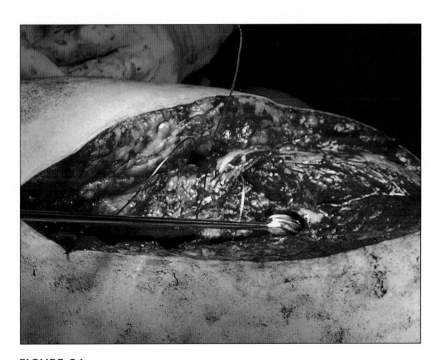

FIGURE 24

- Insert undersized trial stems to get a "feel" for the stability. The final trial is usually slightly smaller than the prosthesis to facilitate removal.
- Check for stability as for primary replacement.
- Insert the definitive component and selected head.
- Closure is similar to that for primary hip replacement (Fig. 25A and 25B), but in revision surgery the increased risk of dislocation is even more important.

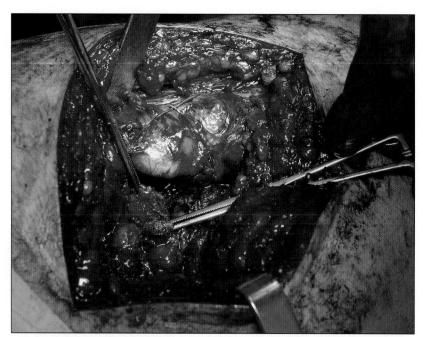

A

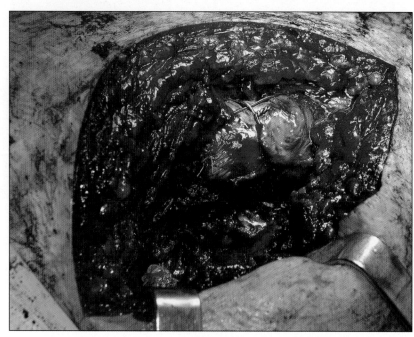

B

FIGURE 25

PEARLS

- Use prophylactic cerclage wire below the defect to prevent fracture.

- Insertion of long stems is easier following an extended trochanteric osteotomy.

- In an intact femur, start with the stem in 90° of anteversion. During impaction, correct this to the normal 15° of anteversion. Anteversion is determined as for primary hip replacement using the axis of the thigh and leg (Fig. 26).

- Chronic stem retroversion during loosening creates a void in the posterior calcar (Fig. 27), making femoral neck geometry unreliable in determining version. Bone graft can fill these defects after definitive stem insertion (Fig. 28).

- Choosing a prosthesis with a high femoral offset increases hip stability.

- If the femoral component will not go down, remove and ream one size larger.

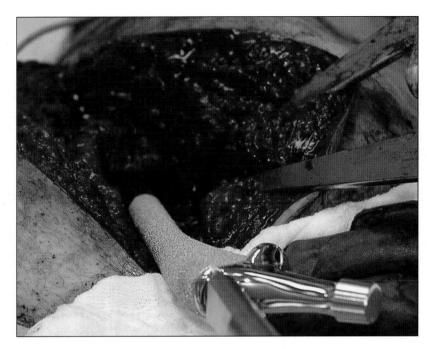

FIGURE 26

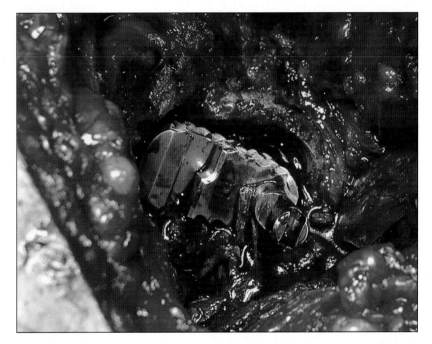

FIGURE 27

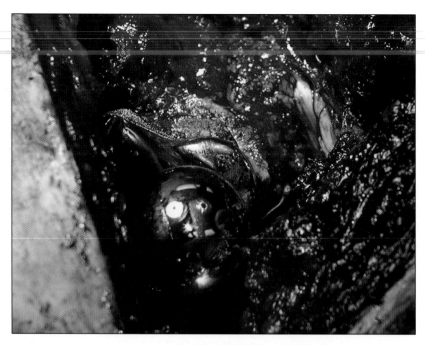

FIGURE 28

PITFALLS

• *Fractures of the femur can occur.*

■ *Undisplaced fractures of the greater trochanter can usually be fixed with a simple figure-of-eight heavy cerclage wire passed around the femur inferior to the lesser trochanter and behind the insertion of the gluteus medius (Fig. 29; see also Fig. 25A and 25B)*

■ *Displaced greater trochanteric fractures require more substantial fixation with cables and a staple or plate (Fig. 30).*

■ *Fractures of the shaft can be treated with a longer bypass stem or femoral strut grafts/plates or a combination (Fig. 31).*

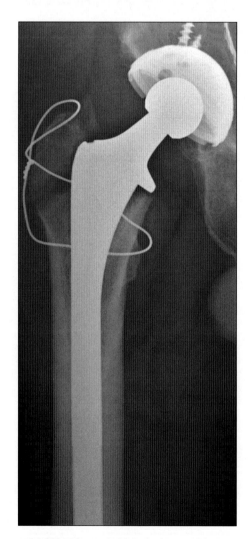

FIGURE 29

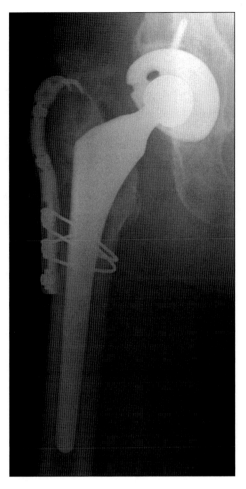

FIGURE 30

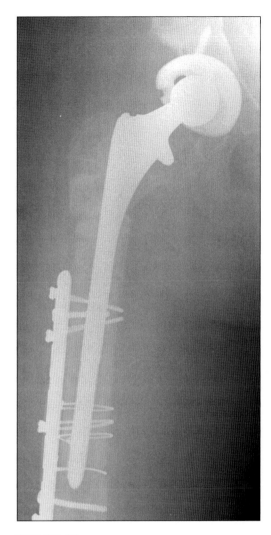

FIGURE 31

Postoperative Care and Expected Outcomes

- Weight bearing is determined by fixation of the femoral stem.
- Possible complications include thromboembolism and heterotrophic ossification.
- Antibiotic prophylaxis is instituted.

Evidence

Engh CA Jr., Ellis TJ, Koralewicz LM, McAuley JP, Engh CA Sr. Extensively porous-coated femoral revision for severe femoral bone loss: minimum 10-year follow-up. J Arthroplasty. 2002;17:955–60.

Whiteside LA. Major femoral bone loss in revision total hip arthroplasty treated with tapered, porous-coated stems. Clin Orthop Relat Res. 2004;(429):222–6.

Two reports of extensive porous coated femoral stems used in the treatment of severe proximal femoral bone loss report good results for stem survival with revision rates of 2.2% (mean follow-up of 38 months) and 89% survival (at a minimum of ten years).

Meneghini RM, Hallab NJ, Berger RA, Jacobs JJ, Paprosky WG, Rosenberg AG. Stem diameter and rotational stability in revision total hip arthroplasty: a biomechanical analysis. J Orthop Surg. 2006;1:5.

A cadaveric study, measuring implant stability in a model bypassing the proximal femur, concluded that larger diameter stems may offer improved stability where the length of diaphyseal contact was short, and that a minimum of 3–4 cm of diaphyseal contact is desirable in cases of proximal femoral bone deficiency.

Moreland JR, Moreno MA. Cementless femoral revision arthroplasty of the hip: minimum 5 years follow-up. Clin Orthop Relat Res. 2001;(393):194–201.

Paprosky WG, Greidanus NV, Antoniou J. Minimum 10-year-results of extensively porous-coated stems in revision hip arthroplasty. Clin Orthop Relat Res. 1999;(369):230–42.

In reviews of 170 and 137 cases (revised with extensive porous coated femoral prostheses), survivorship was reported as 95% at 10 years and as 93% at a mean of 9.3 year follow-up.

INDEX

Note: Page numbers followed by f refer to figures.